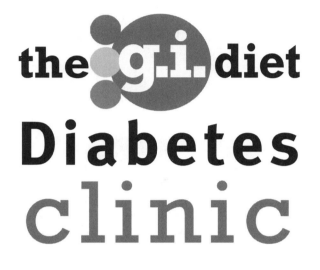

the g.i. diet

Diabetes
clinic

Also by Rick Gallop

the g.i. diet

Diabetes

clinic

RICK GALLOP

RANDOM HOUSE CANADA

Copyright © 2010 Green Light Foods Inc.

All rights reserved under International and Pan-American Copyright Conventions. No part of this book may be reproduced in any form or by any electronic or mechanical means, including information storage and retrieval systems, without permission in writing from the publisher, except by a reviewer, who may quote brief passages in a review. Published in 2010 by Random House Canada, a division of Random House of Canada Limited. Distributed in Canada by Random House of Canada Limited.

Random House Canada and colophon are trademarks.
www.randomhouse.ca

Library and Archives Canada Cataloguing in Publication

Gallop, Rick
    The G.I. diet diabetes clinic : a week-by-week guide to reversing diabetes / Rick Gallop.

Includes index.
ISBN 978–0-307–35709–0

1. Diabetes—Diet therapy. 2. Glycemic index. 3. Reducing diets. I. Title.

RC662.G35 2010 616.4'620654 C2009–905251–2

Printed and bound in Canada

10 9 8 7 6 5 4 3 2 1

*This book is dedicated to the thousands of diabetic readers
who have written to me about their success with the G.I. Diet.
I am particularly grateful to the thirty-seven people
who volunteered for the diabetes e-clinic.
Much of this book is based on their experience.*

Contents

Foreword

I am a family physician in rural New Brunswick where I have practised for over thirty-one years. I have, probably out of necessity because of the huge increase in the number of diabetics in my practice, developed an interest in diabetes. You cannot imagine the excitement I felt when I learned that Rick was writing a G.I. Diet book for Type 2 diabetics. Having seen the marvellous benefits of his other books, I have no doubt whatsoever that his new book will be a major help to anyone living with Type 2 diabetes. And I know that I will be recommending this book to my diabetic patients.

A colleague of mine first introduced me to Rick's books and once I discovered what great tools they were, I did not hesitate to purchase several of them. With my partner Joyce's encouragement, we started this way of life together (it did not feel like a diet) and I experienced tremendous success with weight loss and a significant increase in energy. I started to recommend Rick's books to the overweight and diabetic patients in my medical practice and was pleased to see almost magical results in those who made these dietary changes in their lives. At the time, I had just completed a certification in diabetes and was ready to implement a more aggressive approach with diabetic clients in my medical practice. Without a formal diabetic clinic or a structured diabetic education program in my area, much of this duty fell on family physicians. I worked closely with nurses in the hospital and health care workers from our Extra-Mural Program (a community-based health care service in New Brunswick). I also worked with the one dedicated dietitian at our local hospital who also agreed that the G.I. Diet was highly beneficial for our common patients. Rick's books thus became extremely important for me in counselling my diabetic patients.

It is now well known that overweight and obesity are the principal causes of Type 2 diabetes and pre-diabetes. The G.I. Diet is absolutely ideal for these people because of the dual benefit of both helping them to lose weight as well as stabilizing their blood sugar levels. This disease is so challenging for physicians and diabetic educators but even more so for diabetics themselves. One thing I have learned over the years is that any intervention in the management of diabetes must fit the lifestyle of that person. If health care workers do not tailor the patient's plan to that individual, then suboptimal control of the disease is the end result. Rick's books are so well written, so readable and so easy to follow that I know this new one will easily facilitate the necessary lifestyle changes needed by diabetics to control their disease with a minimum of disruption in their lives.

Thank you, Rick, for caring so much about the health of those struggling with diabetes that you have written this much-needed book.

Dr. William M. Mutrie, B.Sc., M.D.

Introduction

I cannot express how amazing the G.I. Diet has been, I have not only lost 37 pounds to date but I also have been able to manage my blood sugar levels better than I ever had since becoming a diabetic. I have gone from three to four insulin injections a day to two and have been able to go from 24 units per injection to 16. . . . I'm able to enjoy life again without feeling that every-thing is a struggle and exhausting to do. If you follow this diet closely your life and health will truly improve. Believe me because I'm living proof, and God knows I feel WONDERFUL and so ALIVE.
From Cathy, who lost 37 pounds, 7 inches from her waist, and reduced her A1C* from 6.3 to 5.6

All the rules of the G.I. Diet make perfect sense. In my experience, it is the most sensible and safe and healthful approach to weight loss, and it is a way of eating and thinking that can be sustained reasonably for a lifetime. And the thing is, I do believe you don't have to deny yourself the pleasures of eating. . . . Like all endeavours worth doing, the journey is fraught with challenges and hardships, but in the end it's worth it. . . . Now I feel more energetic, I feel encouraged and I feel more in control of my life.
From Kate, who lost 14 pounds, 3 inches from her waist, and reduced her A1C* from 8.0 to 7.2

I love the feeling I get when I see and feel the effects of this clinic . . . I am lighter, happier, healthier, wearing smaller clothing, receiving compliments about my weight loss and can actually feel my ribs and hip bones again !!! What more can I say . . . The scientific and personal support I have received from this experience will enable me to live a healthier and, hopefully, longer life. For that I can't thank you enough.
From Pat, who lost 14 pounds, 2 inches from her waist, and reduced her A1C* from 6.4 to 6.2

* A1C is a measurement of blood sugar levels.

These comments were made by three participants at the conclusion of a 13-week Diabetes e-clinic I recently conducted. If these are the outcomes you would like to see in your life, then this is the book for you. (For a more complete review of the e-clinic results, please turn to page 153.)

Diabetes is rapidly becoming the health epidemic of our new century. In the United States, which unfortunately has become the world's harbinger for disease trends, the incidence of diabetes, especially Type II, has skyrocketed. Pre-diabetes is now designated as an official medical classification, which, if left untreated, invariably leads to full-blown insulin-dependent diabetes.

Here are the latest figures and though these are U.S. statistics, the problem is of a similar magnitude worldwide including developing countries.

Adults with diabetes
    (approximately 70 percent diagnosed: 30 percent undiagnosed) . . . . 10.7 percent
Adults with pre-diabetes . . . . 25.9 percent
Total adults (20 years plus) . . . . 37.6 percent

These figures are staggering and are increasing rapidly. Latest figures show the number of people diagnosed as diabetic or pre-diabetic increased by an astonishing annual rate of 10 percent. Of those diagnosed as diabetic or pre-diabetic, some 90 to 95 percent are Type II or non-insulin-dependent. And of those Type II diabetics or pre-diabetics, 90 percent are overweight or obese. Just to make sure that the magnitude of the problem has sunk in, I'll repeat the key statistic—37.6 percent of the U.S. adult population is diabetic or pre-diabetic.

The principal cause for this rapid increase is insulin resistance. As you are aware, insulin's job is to move sugar (glucose) from the blood into the body's cells for energy and store the surplus as fat. When we overeat, more insulin is produced by the body's pancreatic cells to process the extra sugar. Over time, overeating causes the body's cells that react to the insulin to become overwhelmed by this constant high insulin level and become insulin resistant. This is further compounded by the exhaustion of the pancreatic cells, which are being asked to produce more and more insulin in an attempt to overcome this insulin resistance. Eventually this leads to the perfect diabetic storm—the body's cells becoming increasingly resistant to insulin while the exhausted pancreatic cells decrease insulin production. Either or both outcomes will produce the same result; elevated blood sugar levels leading to Type II diabetes or pre-diabetes.

However, the real villain is overeating, which inevitably leads to being overweight or obese. If that wasn't enough, the extra weight tends to collect around our waistline especially as we reach middle age, which is the typical onset age for Type II diabetes. This is the infamous "apple shape" that both men and women adopt in middle age. This belly fat not only increases insulin resistance but also is associated with other major diseases such as heart disease, hypertension and some forms of cancer.

Though diabetes is dangerous enough in itself to your health, it is also a major contributor to other major diseases. In 68 percent of diabetes-related deaths, 75 percent indicated heart disease as a contributing cause (NIH 2004). Seventy-five percent of diabetic patients reported elevated blood pressure levels. Diabetes is the leading cause of kidney failure; of adult blindness; of non-traumatic lower limb amputations; and there is increasing evidence that it contributes to cognitive impairment. So for those of you who require motivation to get those pounds off, this should be incentive enough.

Obesity is the principal cause of Type II diabetes and pre-diabetes and, unlike many major diseases, it is reversible. Keep in mind that it's you, not the pharmaceutical industry, who can make it happen. The G.I. Diet is the perfect tool. Not only will eating low G.I. green-light foods help stabilize your blood sugar levels, but also you will lose weight. In other words, the G.I. Diet will address both the symptoms—high blood sugar levels—and the root cause—obesity.

So whether you have been diagnosed as Type II diabetic or pre-diabetic, or your doctor advises that you are heading that way unless you lose weight—especially if you have a family history of diabetes—here is your opportunity to save yourself from the deprivations of this dreadful disease and its many life-threatening complications. Just read on.

This book is based on the experiences of a group of thirty-seven men and women diagnosed as diabetic or pre-diabetic who volunteered to participate in a thirteen-week G.I. Diet Diabetes e-clinic. The e-clinic was based on the G.I. Diet, which I originally wrote back in 2002 based on my personal struggle to lose weight when I was president of the Heart and Stroke Foundation of Ontario. The diet I developed is based on the principles of the glycemic index, or G.I., which measures the rate at which the body digests carbohydrates.

The glycemic index was developed in 1980 by a Canadian physician and researcher, Dr. David Jenkins. Early in his career, he became interested in diabetes. At that time, carbohydrates were severely restricted in diabetics' diet because of their potential to boost blood sugar levels, resulting in hypoglycemia. But because the primary role of carbohydrates is to provide the body with energy, diabetics had to make up the lack of calories with a high-fat diet that provided energy without boosting sugar levels. The real quandary was, although diabetics were reducing their risk from hypoglycemia, the high-fat diet increased their risk of heart disease. Dr. Jenkins wondered if all carbohydrates have the same impact on blood sugar levels, or whether some carbohydrates are digested more quickly, thus spiking blood sugar levels. As a result of his research, he published an index—the glycemic index—showing the various rates at which carbohydrates break down, releasing glucose into the blood-stream. The faster the food breaks down, the higher the rating on the index, which sets sugar at 100 and scores all other foods against that number.

Dr. Jenkins also found that his patients were losing weight. Because low-G.I., slow-digesting foods are more satiating, they leave you feeling fuller for a longer period of time. That way you eat less without going hungry, which is the most important criterion for any successful diet. Going hungry is the principal reason that people drop their diets. Low-G.I. foods, such as fruits and vegetables, whole grains, pasta and low-fat dairy products, coupled with lean protein and "best" fats, provide an ideally balanced and nutritious way to eat.

To keep it simple, the G.I. Diet has colour-coded foods into three traffic-light colours. You will never have to count calories or points or weigh and measure food again.

Since the original *G.I. Diet* book hit the shelves, I've heard from tens of thousands of people who are thrilled with their weight loss on the program. Diabetics in particular appeared to have great success losing weight, lowering blood sugar levels and reducing their medication. But as well as hearing about successes, I also heard a lot about readers' challenges and frustrations. Many were coming to the G.I. Diet after a long string of other attempts to manage their weight; having tried every diet under the sun and still failing time and time again. This was particularly true for diabetics who, though they have more motivation than most to change their lifestyle, had in many cases given up hope of ever being able to get their weight back under control.

The dilemma I faced, as do all authors, was that books are, by their nature, a monologue or a one-way communication: I discuss the diet, tell the readers what to do, and that's it—end of story. But these diabetics needed not a monologue—but a dialogue. I had gained some valuable insights into building an interactive experience in two earlier e-clinics; the first dealing with "big people" with serious weight problems; the second with menopausal and postmenopausal women coping with weight gain and other hormonal changes and symptoms. Through the e-clinic, we were able to build an ongoing dialogue as they went through the process of losing weight.

That experience provided me with a template for an e-clinic designed specifically for men and women designated as diabetic or pre-diabetic. The concept was simple: start with the already user-friendly G.I. Diet, and make it even *more* user-friendly by leading participants in detail through the first thirteen critical weeks. During this time, participants were coached on the multiple components of the program: how to handle crises such as falling off the wagon or getting stuck on a weight plateau; and most importantly how to stay motivated—even in the face of unexpected weight gain or cravings for fattening foods. Sticking to the plan was made even easier with complete meal plans covering every meal—and snack—of every day, accompanied by recipes and shopping lists.

In addition, we shared together our day-to-day challenges and discussed solutions as a group. This was conducted by way of weekly communication: I sent to the group a newsletter addressing a particular concern commonly faced by people on the G.I. Diet. In return, once a week each participant sent me their weight and measurements, and a weekly diary illustrating any questions or concerns encountered over the course of the clinic. I reviewed and highlighted some of the issues raised in the participants' diaries and incorporated them into the weekly electronic newsletters.

Though hundreds of people applied for the e-clinic, I chose only thirty-seven to participate. Impressively, especially given the random selection of volunteers, over 90 percent of the group completed the thirteen-week program. This book is a reproduction of the e-clinic that I conducted with these participants. You'll share the same experiences they did: the same menus, the same advice, most likely the same kinds of highs and lows, and—ultimately—the same success.

HOW TO USE THIS BOOK

In **Part I**, I explain the principles of health and nutrition, the basics of successful weight loss, and the way the G.I. Diet works. It's not complicated at all: all foods are traffic-light colour coded:

Red-light—foods to avoid
Yellow-light—foods that you should use occasionally
Green-light—foods you can eat freely

Also included is information on how to make sensible decisions when shopping, cooking, or reading a food label.

Part I deals with nutrition and the mechanics of weight loss, which are critical to your success, I recommend that you read Part I closely before moving on, and refer back to it constantly over the course of your clinic. With a complete understanding of what is happening in your body while you are on the G.I. Diet, you will greatly enhance your chances of success. Don't worry—this isn't rocket science; this is everyday information that's sensible and easy to follow.

Part II is the heart of the matter. Here you'll find the thirteen-week G.I. Diet Diabetes Clinic broken down into week-by-week chapters. Each chapter deals with a different core aspect of success on the G.I. Diet—matters such as behaviour change, staying motivated, and how to keep your diet intact when eating out, as well as issues pertaining to diabetes.

As this book is primarily concerned with weight loss, we do not propose to make this a primer on diabetes. However, should you require additional material about diabetes, I have found *The Diabetes Sourcebook* by doctors Diana and Richard Guthrie to be a good source as it contains both the latest information and—more importantly—information that can be understood by the non-medical reader. The best overall web-based source is the National Diabetes Information Clearinghouse provided by the U.S. National Institute of Health: www.diabetol.niddk.nih.gov. An excellent Canadian website is the Canadian Diabetes Association at www.diabetes.ca.

Whether you are currently pre-diabetic or fully diagnosed, the G.I. Diet Diabetes Clinic will help you regain your waistline and energy levels, and improve your health. My discussion of each topic is accompanied by what the participants of the original e-clinic had to say about these subjects as well as their own experiences.

Each week I include readers' diabetes-related success stories from the thousands of letters I have received, so you can see how the G.I. Diet worked for them, as well as the lessons they learned. I believe you will find these successes most motivating.

The weekly sequence is laid out in an intentional order that loosely maps the experiences you'll have over the course of three months on the G.I. Diet. Week 1, for instance, is Getting Started; while Week 9 is Staying the Course. However, the clinic is not rigid! If you, for instance, find yourself having difficulties eating out-side your home, reread or skip forward to the appropriate chapter. Of particular note is Week 10, Celebrations: Holidays and Entertaining, which addresses those days and celebrations when we often find it difficult to stick to our healthy eating habits. Of course, visit the advice and recommendations for this week when a holiday or celebration comes up on your calendar—move it up a few weeks, or push it back, as necessary.

Each week also includes a page reference to a detailed meal plan (three daily meals, plus snacks) located in Part IV. Along with the meal plan you will find an accompanying grocery list that lists all you need to make the week's worth of food. These meal plans are both optional and flexible and repeat over weeks 5 through 13—a note at the end of each week tells you to which meal plan you should refer. While some people who prefer a fully structured program might follow each day to the letter, others might prefer to plan their own green-light meals and snacks, using the meal plan only as a guide. Diary space is provided for you to record your measurements and your observations or comments on your weekly experience with the diet and your changing lifestyle.

Part III deals with life after the first thirteen weeks, both for those who have reached their target weight and for those who still have some way to go. This section outlines Phase II of the G.I. Diet, reintroducing some yellow-light treats, modify-ing your diet as you approach your target weight, and providing advice on eating in order to maintain your new healthy weight for the rest of your life.

Once you've made it through the thirteen weeks outlined in this book, you are invited to sign on for nine monthly e-mail newsletters, which will provide you with support, the latest news on green-light products and dishes, and further recipes and tips. An on-line Green-Light Discussion Forum is also available. I also invite you to submit your own monthly diary and measurements in response to these letters—an ongoing e-clinic of your very own! See page 153 for more information on this program.

Part IV begins with four basic meal plans (with grocery lists) that rotate through the weeks. Following the meal plans, I have listed over seventy delicious recipes divided by meal type—virtually all the recipes you'll need in order to make the dishes suggested in each week's meal plan. The recipes are green-light, low-G.I., and (best of all) delicious—you'll know you've made the right choice of diet when you try the recipe for Pecan Brownies (page 269)!

The recipes are followed by a comprehensive breakdown of common foods and ingredients, categorizing the contents into the three traffic-light colours—red, yellow, and green. It's a handy reference for times when your palate wanders from the meals and recipes indicated elsewhere in the book. Copy it and take it with you when eating out, especially in the first month of the program when you are making adjustments to your eating habits. Whether you are diabetic or pre-diabetic, and whether this is your first introduction to the G.I. Diet program, or you are an old hand looking for a new approach, I'm confident that this clinic will help you lose weight permanently, lower your blood sugar levels and reduce your medication dependency. This is not so much a diet as a new way of eating that allows you to lose weight without going hungry or feeling deprived. The traffic-light colour coding of foods keeps it simple so you'll never have to count another calorie. And, finally, it's a balanced, nutritious diet that will help you reduce the risk of major diseases and live a longer and more active life.

PART I : The G.I. Diet

Chapter One
The Truth about Carbs, Fats and Protein

It's just about impossible to live in this country and not know that we are in the midst of an "obesity epidemic." If you watch television, listen to the radio, read the newspaper or simply notice the magazine headlines at the supermarket checkout, you can't help but be aware that nearly 56 percent of Canadians are overweight and that our obesity rate has doubled over the past twenty years. Everyone seems to have an explanation for our collective weight crisis: some hold the fast-food industry responsible; others blame our sedentary lifestyle. Some maintain we are eating too much fat; others say we are eating too many carbohydrates. So what's the truth?

Well, all of these reasons are part of the answer. But if you reduce the problem to its physiological cause, it's actually quite simple: we're consuming more calories than we're expending, and the resulting surplus is stored around our waists, hips and thighs as fat. There's no mystery here. But to understand why we are consuming more calories, we need to get back to basics and look at the three fundamental elements of our diet: carbohydrates, fats and protein. We need to understand the role these components play in the digestive system and how they work together—whether we're in the process of getting fat or thin.

We'll start with carbohydrates, since the popularity of low-carbohydrate diets like the Atkins program has made them a hot topic and given them a bad rap. Carbohydrates have been so much in the news over the past few years that a new word—"carbs"—has entered the language. Though they've been blamed for all our weight problems, their role in weight control has really been misunderstood.

CARBOHYDRATES
Carbohydrates are a necessary part of a healthy diet. They are rich in fibre, vitamins and minerals, including antioxidants, which we now know play an important role in the prevention of heart disease and cancer. Carbohydrates are also the primary

source of energy for our bodies. They are found in grains, vegetables, fruits, legumes (beans) and dairy products.

Here is how carbs work: when you eat an orange or a bagel, your body digests the carbohydrates in the food and turns them into glucose, which provides you with energy. The glucose dissolves in your bloodstream and then travels to the parts of your body that use energy, such as your muscles and brain. So carbs are critical to everyone's health. When managing weight, however, it is important to realize that not all carbs are created equal.

Some carbohydrates break down into glucose in the digestive system at a slow and steady rate, gradually releasing their nutrients and keeping us feeling full and satisfied. Others break down rapidly, spiking our glucose levels and then disappearing quickly, leaving us feeling hungry again. For example, cornflakes and old-fashioned, large-flake oatmeal are both carbohydrates, but we all know the difference between eating a bowl of oatmeal for breakfast and eating a bowl of cornflakes. The oatmeal stays with you—it "sticks to your ribs," as my mother used to say—whereas your stomach starts rumbling an hour after eating the cornflakes, pushing you toward your next snack or meal. Throughout the course of a day, if you are eating carbs that break down rapidly, like cornflakes, as opposed to those that break down slowly, you will be eating more and, as a result, will begin to put on weight. If, however, you start eating carbs that break down slowly, like old-fashioned oatmeal, you will eat less and begin to lose weight. Selecting the right type of carb is key to achieving your optimum energy and weight. But how do you know which carbohydrate is the right type and which isn't?

Well, the first clue is the amount of processing that the food has undergone. The more a food is processed beyond its natural, fibrous state, the less processing your body has to do to digest it. The quicker you digest the food, the sooner you feel hungry again. This helps explain why the number of Canadian adults who are over-weight has surged over the last fifty years. A hundred years ago, most of the food people ate came straight from the farm to the dinner table. Lack of refrigeration and scant knowledge of food chemistry meant that most food remained in its original state. However, advances in science, along with the migration of many women out of the kitchen and into the workforce, led to a revolution in prepared foods geared to speed and simplicity of preparation. The giant food companies—Kraft, Kellogg's, Del Monte, Nestlé, etc.—were born. We happily began spending more money for the convenience of prepared, processed, packaged, canned, frozen and bottled food. The Kraft Dinner era had begun.

It was during this period that the miller's traditional wind and water mills were replaced with high-speed steel rolling mills, which stripped away most of the key nutrients, including the bran, fibre and wheat germ (which could spoil), to produce a talcum-like powder: today's white flour. This fine white flour is the basic ingredient for most of our breads and cereals, as well as for baked goods and snacks such as cookies, muffins, crackers and pretzels. Walk through any supermarket and you will be surrounded by towering stacks of these flour-based processed products. And we're eating more and more of these foods; over the past three decades our consumption of grain has increased by 50 percent. Our bodies are paying the price for this radical change in eating habits.

The second clue in determining whether a carbohydrate is the right type is the amount of fibre it contains. Fibre, in simple terms, provides low-calorie filler. It does double duty, in fact: it literally fills up your stomach, so you feel satiated; and your body takes much longer to break it down, so it stays with you longer and slows the digestive process. There are two forms of fibre: soluble and insoluble. Soluble fibre is found in carbs such as oatmeal, beans, barley and citrus fruits, and has been shown to lower blood cholesterol levels. Insoluble fibre is important for normal bowel function and is typically found in whole wheat breads and cereals, and most vegetables.

There are two other important components that inhibit the rapid breakdown of food in our digestive system, and they are fats and protein. Let's look at fats first.

FATS

Fat, like fibre, acts as a brake in the digestive process. When combined with other foods, fat becomes a barrier to digestive juices. It also signals the brain that you are satisfied and do not require more food. Does this mean that we should eat all the fat we want? Definitely not!

Though fat is essential for a nutritious diet, containing various key elements that are crucial to the digestive process, cell development and overall health, it also contains twice the number of calories per gram as carbohydrates and protein. If you decide to "just add peanut butter" to your otherwise disciplined regime, it doesn't take much of it—two tablespoons—to turbo-charge your total calorie count. As well, once you eat fat, your body is a genius at hanging onto it and refusing to let it go. This occurs because fat is how the body stores reserve supplies of energy, usually around the waist, hips and thighs. Fat is money in the bank as far as the body is concerned— a rainy-day investment for when you have to call up extra energy. This clever system originally helped our ancestors survive during periods of famine. The problem today is that we don't live with cycles of feast and famine—it's more like feast, and then feast again! But the body's eagerness for fat continues, along with its reluctance to give it up.

This is why losing weight is so difficult: your body does everything it can to persuade you to eat more fat. How? Through fat's capacity to make things taste good. So it's not just you who thinks that juicy steaks, chocolate cake and rich ice cream taste better than a bean sprout. That's the fat content of cake and steak talking.

Sorry to say, there's no getting around it: if you want to lose weight, you have to watch your fat consumption. In addition, you need to be concerned about the type of fats you eat; many fats are harmful to your health. There are four types of fat: the best, the good, the bad and the really ugly. The "really ugly" fats are potentially the most dangerous, and they lurk in many of our most popular snack foods. They are vegetable oils that have been heat-treated to make them thicken—the trans fats you've been hearing so much about in the media. They raise the amount of LDL, or bad, cholesterol in our bodies while lowering the amount of HDL, or good, cholesterol, which protects us from heart disease. As a result, they boost our cholesterol levels, which thickens our arteries and causes heart attack and stroke. So avoid using trans fats, such as vegetable shortening and hard margarine, and avoid packaged snack foods, baked goods, crackers and cereals that contain them. (You can spot them by checking labels for "hydrogenated" or "partially hydrogenated" oils.)

The "bad" fats are called saturated fats and almost always come from animal sources. Butter, cheese and meat are all high in saturated fats. There are a couple of others you should be aware of too: coconut oil and palm oil are two vegetable oils that are saturated and, because they are cheap, they are used in many snack foods, especially cookies. Saturated fats, such as butter or cheese, are solid at room temperature. They elevate your risk of heart disease and Alzheimer's. The evidence is also growing that many cancers, including colon, prostate and breast cancer, are associated with diets high in saturated fats.

The "good" fats are the polyunsaturated and monounsaturated ones, which are cholesterol free. Most vegetable oils, such as corn and sunflower, fall into this category. What you really should be eating, however, are the "best" fats, the monounsaturated fats, which actually promote good health. These are the fats found in olives, almonds, and canola and olive oils. Monounsaturated fats have a beneficial effect on cholesterol and are good for your heart. This is one reason the incidence of heart disease is low in Mediterranean countries, where olive oil is a staple. Although fancy olive oil is expensive, you can enjoy the same health benefits from less costly supermarket brands.

Another highly beneficial oil that falls into the "best" category is omega-3, a fatty acid found in deep-sea fish, such as salmon, mackerel, albacore tuna and herring, as well as in lake trout, walnuts, and flaxseed and canola oils. Some brands of eggs and liquid eggs also contain omega-3, which can help lower cholesterol and protect cardiovascular health.

So the "best" and "good" fats are an important part of a healthy diet and also help slow digestion. Still, they're fat and they pack a lot of calories. Over twice as many calories per gram as carbohydrates or protein. We have to be careful, then, to limit our intake of these polyunsaturated and monounsaturated fats when trying to lose weight.

Since protein also acts as a brake in the digestive process, let's look at it in more detail.

PROTEIN

Protein is an absolutely essential part of your diet. In fact, you are already half protein: 50 percent of your dry body weight is made up of muscles, organs, skin and hair, all forms of protein. We need this element to build and repair body tissues, and it figures in nearly all metabolic reactions. Protein is also a critical brain food, providing amino acids for the neurotransmitters that relay messages to the brain. This is why it's not a good idea to skip breakfast on the morning of a big meeting or exam. The "brain fog" people experience on some diets is likely the result of diminished protein. Protein is literally food for thought.

The main sources of dietary protein come from animals: meat, seafood, dairy and eggs. Vegetable sources include beans and soy-based products such as tofu. Unfortunately, protein sources such as red meat and full-fat dairy products are also high in "bad," or saturated, fats, which are harmful to your health. It is important that we get our protein from sources that are low in saturated fats, such as lean meats, skinless poultry, seafood, low-fat dairy products, cholesterol-reduced liquid eggs, and tofu and other soy products. One exceptional source of protein is the humble bean. Beans are a perfect food, really: they're high in protein and fibre, and low in saturated fat. No wonder so many of the world's cuisines have found myriad wonderful ways to cook beans. North Americans need to become more bean savvy.

Nuts are another excellent source of protein and are relatively low in fat—as long as you don't eat a whole bowlful.

Protein is much more effective than carbohydrates or fat at satisfying hunger. It will make you feel fuller longer, which is why you should try to incorporate some protein into every meal and snack. This will help keep you on the ball and feeling satisfied.

Now that we know how carbohydrates, fats and protein work in the digestive system, let's use the science to discover how to take off the extra pounds.

TO SUM UP

- Eat carbohydrates that have not been highly processed and that do not contain highly processed ingredients.
- Eat less fat overall and look for low-fat alternatives to your current food choices.
- Eat only monounsaturated and polyunsaturated fats.
- Include some protein, preferably from both animal and vegetable sources.

Chapter Two
The Secret to Easy, Permanent Weight Loss

While most people reading this are diabetic or pre-diabetic, and therefore familiar with the glycemic index and its impact on blood sugar levels, I thought a recap might be helpful for those of you who have more recently been diagnosed. It is important that everybody have a basic knowledge about the glycemic index as it is critical to understanding this diet.

The "G.I." in G.I. Diet stands for Glycemic Index, which is the basis of this diet—and the only scientific phrase you'll need to know. The glycemic index is the secret to reducing calories and losing weight without going hungry. It measures the speed at which carbohydrates break down in our digestive system and turn into glucose, the body's main source of energy or fuel.

In the Introduction I provided some information as to how Dr. David Jenkins developed the glycemic index. In short, he found that certain carbohydrates broke down quickly and flooded the bloodstream with sugar, but others broke down more slowly, only marginally increasing blood sugar levels. The faster a food breaks down, the higher its rating on the glycemic index, which sets sugar at 100 and scores all other foods against that number. These findings were important to diabetics, who could then use the index to identify low–G.I., slow-release foods that would help control their blood sugar levels. At right are some examples of the G.I. ratings of a range of popular foods.

What do these G.I. ratings have to do with the numbers on your bathroom scale? Well, it turns out that low–G.I., slow-release foods have a significant impact on our ability to lose weight. As I have explained, when we eat the wrong type of carb, a high–G.I. food, the body quickly digests it and releases a flood of sugar (glucose) into the

EXAMPLES OF G.I. RATINGS			
HIGH G.I.		LOW G.I.	
Baguette	95	Orange	44
Cornflakes	84	All-Bran	43
Rice Cake	82	Oatmeal	42
Doughnut	76	Spaghetti	41
Bagel	72	Apple	38
Cereal bar	72	Beans	31
Biscuit	69	Plain yogurt	25

bloodstream. This gives us a short-term high, but the sugar is just as quickly absorbed by the body, leaving us with a post-sugar slump. We feel lethargic and start looking for our next sugar fix. A fast-food lunch of a double cheeseburger, fries and a Coke delivers a short-term burst of energy, but by mid-afternoon we start feeling tired, sluggish and hungry. That's when we reach for "just one" brownie or bag of potato chips. These high–G.I. foods deliver the rush we want and then let us down again. The roller-coaster ride is a hard cycle to break. But a high–G.I. diet will make you feel hungry more often, so you end up eating more and gaining more weight.

Let's look at the other end of the G.I. index. Low–G.I. foods, such as fruits, vegetables, whole grains, pasta, beans and low-fat dairy products, take longer to digest, deliver a steady supply of sugar to our bloodstream and leave us feeling fuller for a longer time. Consequently, we eat less. It also helps that these foods are lower in calories. As a result, we consume less food and fewer calories, without going hungry or feeling unsatisfied.

The key player in this process of energy storage and retrieval is insulin, a hormone secreted by the pancreas. Insulin does two things very well. First, as you are aware, it regulates the amount of sugar (glucose) in our bloodstream, removing the excess and storing it as glycogen for immediate use by our muscles, or putting it into storage as fat. Second, insulin acts as a security guard at the fat gates, reluctantly giving up its reserves. This evolutionary feature is a throwback to the days when our ancestors were hunter-gatherers, habitually experiencing times of feast or famine. When food was in abundance, the body stored its surplus as fat to tide it over the inevitable days of famine.

A few years ago, I was on vacation in a remote part of central Mexico, visiting the Copper Canyon, which, incredibly, is larger and deeper than the Grand Canyon in Arizona. A tribe of Tarahumara Indians still resides there. Until recently, these indigenous peoples typically put on 30 pounds during the summer and fall, when the crops, particularly corn, were plentiful. Then, over the course of the winter, when food became scarce, they lost these 30 pounds. Insulin was the champion in this process, both helping to accumulate fat and then guarding its depletion.

Of course, food is now readily available to us at the nearest twenty-four-hour supermarket. But our bodies still function very much as they did in the earliest days. When we eat a high–G.I. food, our pancreas releases insulin to reduce the glucose level in our blood, which, if left unchecked, would lead to hyperglycemia. If we aren't using all that energy at the moment, the glucose is stored as fat. Soon we become hungry again. Our body can either draw on our reserves of fat and laboriously convert them back to sugar, or it can look for more food. Since giving up extra fat is the body's last choice—who knows when that supply might come in handy?—our body would rather send us to the fridge than work to convert fat back to sugar. This helped our survival back in the old days, but it gets in the way of weight loss now.

Blood sugar levels are also influenced by hormonal changes. For women, your period, pregnancy and menopause all create hormonal swings that cause blood sugar levels to fluctuate. This is a principal trigger for weight, as well as changes in mood—PMS is a classic example. With menopause, these hormonal changes are more extreme and long lasting. They result in not only weight gain and mood swings, but also other menopausal symptoms such as interrupted sleep patterns and hot flashes. Stabilizing your blood sugar levels will go a long way to help manage these symptoms, and the G.I. Diet can help.

So our goal is to limit the amount of insulin in our system by avoiding high–G.I. foods, which stimulate its production, and instead choosing low–G.I. foods, which keep the supply of sugar in our bloodstream consistent. Slow-release, low–G.I. carbohydrates help curb your appetite by leaving you feeling fuller for a longer period of time. When you combine them with lean protein and the best fats, which help slow the digestive process, you have the magic combination that will allow you to lose weight without going hungry.

For diabetics, this provides a double benefit. First you lose weight, the root cause of your diabetes. And second, by lowering and stabilizing your blood sugar levels, you are better able to control the symptoms. As we will see, three-quarters of those on medication in the e-clinic were able to reduce their medication over the thirteen-week program.

Translated into real food, what does this mean? Well, for dinner you could have a grilled chicken breast, boiled new potatoes, a side salad of romaine lettuce and red pepper dressed with a bit of olive oil and lemon juice, and some asparagus if you feel like it. The trick is to stick with foods that have a low G.I., are low in fat and are lowish in calories. This sounds—and is, in fact—quite complex. It might seem to you as though I'm breaking my promise of an easy weight-loss plan. But don't worry: I've done all the calculations, measurements and math for you, and sorted the foods you like to eat into one of three categories based on the colours of the traffic light. On pages 271–277, you will find the Complete G.I. Diet Food Guide, which has a list of foods in a red column, a list in a yellow column and a list in a green column. Here's how the colour-coded categories work:

RED-LIGHT FOODS

The foods in the red column are to be avoided. They are high–G.I., higher-calorie foods that will make it impossible for you to lose weight.

YELLOW-LIGHT FOODS

The foods in the yellow column are mid-range G.I. foods that should be treated with caution. They should be avoided when you are trying to lose weight, but once you've slimmed down to your ideal weight, you can begin to enjoy yellow-light foods from time to time.

GREEN-LIGHT FOODS

The green column lists foods that are low–G.I., low in fat and lower in calories. These are the foods that will allow you to lose weight. Don't expect them to be taste-less and boring! There are many delicious and satisfying choices that will make you feel as though you aren't even on a diet.

If you're a veteran of the low-carbohydrate craze, you'll be surprised to find pota-toes and rice in the green-light column, but they are fine as long as they are the right type. Baked potatoes and french fries have a high G.I., while boiled new potatoes have a lower G.I. The short-grain, glutinous rice served in Chinese and Thai restaurants is high–G.I., while long-grain, brown, basmati and wild rice are low. Pasta is also a green-light food—as long as it is cooked only until al dente (with some firmness to the bite). Any processing of food, including cooking, increases a food's G.I., since heat breaks down starch capsules and fibre, giving your digestive juices a head start. This is why you should never overcook vegetables; instead, steam them or microwave them in a small amount of water just until they are tender. This way, they will retain their vitamins and other nutrients, and their G.I. rating will remain low.

While eating green-light foods is really the core of the G.I. Diet, there are a few more things you'll need to know to follow the program. Let's discuss these in the next chapter.

TO SUM UP
- Low–G.I foods take longer to digest, so you feel satiated longer.
- The key to losing weight is to eat low–G.I., low-calorie foods—in other words, foods from the green-light column of the Complete G.I. Diet Food Guide.

Chapter Three
The G.I. Diet Essentials

The G.I. Diet consists of two phases. For those with a more serious weight problem, an additional Preliminary Phase has been added. The Preliminary Phase and Phase I are the dramatic parts of the G.I. Diet—the period when those extra unwanted pounds come off! During these stages, you'll focus on eating foods that are low–G.I. and also low in fat and sugar—the foods in the green-light column of the Complete G.I. Diet Food Guide on pages 271–277. Yes, this means a farewell to bagels and a fond adieu to Häagen-Dazs. But it doesn't mean you won't have a multitude of delicious foods to choose from. Once you've slimmed down to your ideal weight, you enter Phase II, the maintenance phase of the program, which is the way you will eat for the rest of your life.

To decide whether you will be starting with the Preliminary Phase or Phase I, you will need to find out your body mass index (BMI), which is a measurement of how much body fat you are carrying relative to your height.

YOUR BMI

While the BMI gives a relatively accurate measure of body fat, it applies only to people who are twenty to sixty-five years of age. It isn't valid for children, pregnant or nursing women, the elderly or heavily muscled athletes. For the rest of us, however, it is the only accepted international standard for weight.

You can calculate your BMI from the table on pages 26–27 by running your finger down the left vertical column of the table until you reach your height. Then run your finger across that row until you find the number that is closest to your weight. The number at the top of that column is your BMI.

If your BMI falls between 19 and 24, your weight is within the acceptable norm and is considered healthy. Anything between 25 and 29 is considered overweight; if you're 30 or over, you are officially obese. If your BMI is 32 or under, I recommend you begin with Phase I of the program. If it's over 32, then start with the Preliminary Phase.

FRAME SIZE

You will note that the BMI tables have a broad range of weights in each of the weight categories—healthy weight (BMI 19–24), overweight (BMI 25–29) and obese (BMI 30 and over). A 5'5" woman, for instance, has a healthy weight range from 114 pounds (BMI 19) to 144 pounds (BMI 24). The reason for this broad range is primarily to allow for variances in people's different frame sizes.

People with small frames should have a healthy weight in the bottom third of the range while those with large frames, in the top third; (i.e., small frame, BMI 19–21; medium frame, BMI 21–22; large frame, BMI 23–24).

To calculate which size frame you fit into, here is a guide for **women** based on your wrist measurement. The measurement should be taken with a tape measure at the narrowest point on your wrist.

WRIST SIZE IN INCHES	HEIGHT UNDER 5'2"	HEIGHT 5'2"-5'5"	HEIGHT OVER 5'5"
Under 5.50	S	S	S
5.50–5.75	M	S	S
5.75–6.00	L	S	S
6.00–6.25	L	M	S
6.25–6.50	L	L	M
Over 6.50	L	L	L

Key:
S = Small frame
M = Medium frame
L = Large frame
Source: National Library of Medicine

So Diane, who is 5'7" and has a wrist measurement of 6.0 inches, will have a small frame. Her healthy weight will therefore be between 121 and 127 pounds (BMI 19–20). Jennifer, on the other hand, who is also 5'7", has a wrist measurement of 6.6 inches and therefore has a large frame. Jennifer's healthy weight, by comparison, will range from 146 to 153 pounds (BMI 23–24) or 25 pounds more than Diane's.

For **men** who are 5'5" or more, then your measurements are simply:

Wrist under 6.5 inches = small frame
Wrist 6.5–7.5 inches = medium frame
Wrist over 7.5 inches = large frame

THE PRELIMINARY PHASE AND PHASE I

To determine whether to begin with the Preliminary Phase or with Phase I, take a look at the BMI chart. If your BMI is 32 or under, I recommend you begin with Phase I of the program. If your BMI is over 32, start with the Preliminary Phase. The Preliminary Phase is, in effect, a "step-in" plan that helps reduce any initial hunger pangs caused by a sudden drop in calories that people with a significant weight problem sometimes experience.

The Preliminary Phase lasts as long as you continue to weigh more than 32 on the BMI chart. So it is important that you recalculate your BMI when you weigh yourself every week. If you feel that you can manage without the Preliminary Phase, please feel free to go straight to Phase I. About half of the original "big-people" e-clinic members with a BMI of over 32 elected to do this without significant difficulty.

Now that you know whether you'll be starting with the Preliminary Phase or Phase I, it's time to get into the details: what to eat, how much and how often.

WHAT DO I EAT?

As you know, during the Preliminary Phase and Phase I, you will be sticking to the foods listed in the green-light column of the Complete G.I. Diet Food Guide on pages 271–277. To get a breakdown of your green-light choices for each meal, turn to pages 28–29(breakfast), 32–34 (lunch), 35–37 (dinner) and 40–41 (snacks).

HOW MUCH DO I EAT?

Remember, this is not a starvation diet—far from it. Going hungry is simply not necessary for weight loss; in fact, it's something to be resolutely avoided! Hunger is the absolute death knell for any weight-loss program. If you are hungry for a sustained period of time, your body will feel that it hasn't received enough fuel to meet its needs and will slow the rate at which it burns calories, making it even harder to lose those extra pounds. So never leave your digestive system with nothing to do. If your digestive system is busy processing food and steadily supplying energy to your brain, not only will your metabolism keep firing at a steady rate, but also you won't be looking for high-calorie snacks. This is why you can, for the most part, eat as much green-light food as you want on the G.I. Diet.

In Phase I, you should be eating three meals and three snacks every day. And in the Preliminary Phase, you should be eating three meals and four snacks every day. The reason I recommend an extra snack in the Preliminary Phase is that someone with a larger body requires more calories just to keep functioning on a daily basis than someone who is lighter. This is also why I suggest larger serving sizes for some green-light foods in the Preliminary Phase than in Phase I. Although I generally do not restrict quantities of green-light foods—within reason (five heads of cabbage is a bit extreme)—there are a few exceptions, which I outline below. (Except where indicated, a serving size is per meal, not per day.)

PORTIONS

Each meal and snack should contain, if possible, a combination of green-light protein, carbohydrates—especially vegetables and fruit—and fats. An easy way to visualize portion size is to divide your plate into three sections (see illustration). Half the plate should be filled with vegetables; one-quarter should contain protein, such as lean meat, poultry, seafood, eggs, tofu or legumes; and the last quarter should contain a green-light serving of rice, pasta or potatoes.

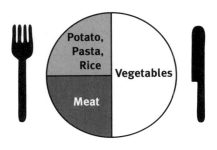

WHEN DO I EAT?

Try to eat regularly throughout the day. If you skimp on breakfast and lunch, you will probably be starving by dinner and end up piling on the food. Have one snack mid-morning, another mid-afternoon and the last before bed. In the Preliminary Phase, the fourth snack can be eaten later in the afternoon if you usually have a late dinner, or during the evening if you generally have an early dinner. It's really up to you—have the extra snack at the time of day when you feel you most need it. The idea is to keep your digestive system happily busy so you won't start craving those red-light snacks.

GREEN-LIGHT SERVINGS

GREEN-LIGHT FOOD	PRELIMINARY PHASE (BMI OF 33 OR MORE)	PHASE I (BMI OF 32 OR LESS)
Crispbreads (with high fibre, e.g., Wasa Fibre)	3 crispbreads	2 crispbreads
Green-light breads (which have at least 2 ½ to 3 grams of fibre per slice)	2 slices per day	1 slice per day
Green-light cereals	²/₃ cup	½ cup
Green-light nuts	12 to 15	8 to 10
Margarine (non-hydrogenated, light)	3 teaspoons	2 teaspoons
Meat, fish, poultry	6 ounces	4 ounces (about the size of a pack of cards)
Olive/canola oil	1 ½ teaspoons	1 teaspoon
Olives	6 to 8	4 to 5
Pasta	1 cup cooked	¾ cup cooked
Potatoes (new or small, boiled)	4 to 5	2 to 3
Rice (basmati, brown, long-grain)	¾ cup cooked	²/₃ cup cooked

BODY MASS

BMI	NORMAL						OVERWEIGHT					OBESE	
	19	20	21	22	23	24	25	26	27	28	29	30	31
HEIGHT	**WEIGHT (POUNDS)**												
4'10"	91	96	100	105	110	115	119	124	129	134	138	143	148
4'11"	94	99	104	109	114	119	124	128	133	138	143	148	153
5'0"	97	102	107	112	118	123	128	133	138	143	148	153	158
5'1"	100	106	111	116	122	127	132	137	143	148	153	158	164
5'2"	104	109	115	120	126	131	136	142	147	153	158	164	169
5'3"	107	113	118	124	130	135	141	146	152	158	163	169	175
5'4"	110	116	122	128	134	140	145	151	157	163	169	174	180
5'5"	114	120	126	132	138	144	150	156	162	168	174	180	186
5'6"	118	124	130	136	142	148	155	161	167	173	179	186	192
5'7"	121	127	134	140	146	153	159	166	172	178	185	191	198
5'8"	125	131	138	144	151	158	164	171	177	184	190	197	203
5'9"	128	135	142	149	155	162	169	176	182	189	196	203	209
5'10"	132	139	146	153	160	167	174	181	188	195	202	209	216
5'11"	136	143	150	157	165	172	179	186	193	200	208	215	222
6'0"	140	147	154	162	169	177	184	191	199	206	213	221	228
6'1"	144	151	159	166	174	182	189	197	204	212	219	227	235
6'2"	148	155	163	171	179	186	194	202	210	218	225	233	241
6'3"	152	160	168	176	184	192	200	208	216	224	232	240	248
6'4"	156	164	172	180	189	197	205	213	221	230	238	246	254

Source: U.S. National Heart, Lung and Blood Institute

INDEX (BMI)

	OBESE							EXTREMELY OBESE					
32	33	34	35	36	37	38	39	40	41	42	43	44	45

WEIGHT (POUNDS)

32	33	34	35	36	37	38	39	40	41	42	43	44	45
153	158	162	167	172	177	181	186	191	196	201	205	210	215
158	163	168	173	178	183	188	193	198	203	208	212	217	222
163	168	174	179	184	189	194	199	204	209	215	220	225	230
169	174	180	185	190	195	201	206	211	217	222	227	232	238
175	180	186	191	196	202	207	213	218	224	229	235	240	246
180	186	191	197	203	208	214	220	225	231	237	242	248	254
186	192	197	204	209	215	221	227	232	238	244	250	256	262
192	198	204	210	216	222	228	234	240	246	252	258	264	270
198	204	210	216	223	229	235	241	247	253	260	266	272	278
204	211	217	223	230	236	242	249	255	261	268	274	280	287
210	216	223	230	236	243	249	256	262	269	276	282	289	295
216	223	230	236	243	250	257	263	270	277	284	291	297	304
222	229	236	243	250	257	264	271	278	285	292	299	306	313
229	236	243	250	257	265	272	279	286	293	301	308	315	322
235	242	250	258	265	272	279	287	294	302	309	316	324	331
242	250	257	265	272	280	288	295	302	310	318	325	333	340
249	256	264	272	280	287	295	303	311	319	326	334	342	350
256	264	272	279	287	295	303	311	319	327	335	343	351	359
263	271	279	287	295	304	312	320	328	336	344	353	361	369

MEAL BASICS

Though most diabetics should be aware of food to avoid, experience with the e-clinic demonstrated a surprising lack of knowledge. So if the low–G.I. green-light way of eating is new to you, you're probably wondering what to eat instead of that bagel with cream cheese for breakfast, that hamburger for lunch and those tortilla chips and salsa for a snack. On the following pages I'll go over your various green-light options for each of the main meals and snacks of your daily G.I. program. Let's start with breakfast.

BREAKFAST

I know you've been told that breakfast is the most important meal of the day, and it's actually true. It's the first thing you eat after your night-long "fast" of twelve hours or more, and it launches you into your workday. Eating a healthy breakfast will help you avoid the need to grab a coffee and Danish as soon as you hit the office, and will make you feel satisfied and energetic. Eating breakfast every day doesn't mean you have to set the alarm any earlier. If you have time to read the paper or feed the cat, you have time to prepare and eat a green-light breakfast.

The following chart lists typical breakfast foods in the colour-coded categories. To ensure you have a balanced breakfast, include some green-light carbohydrates, protein and fat. For a complete list of foods, see the Complete G.I. Diet Food Guide on pages 271–277.

Let's take a closer look at some of the usual breakfast choices.

PROTEIN			
Meat and Eggs	Regular bacon Sausages	Turkey bacon Whole regular eggs (preferable omega-3)	Back bacon Lean ham Liquid eggs/egg whites

Dairy	Cheese
	Cottage cheese (whole
	    or 2%)
	Cream
	Milk (whole or 2%)
	Sour cream
	Yogurt (whole or 2%)
		Cream cheese (light)
		Milk (1%)
		Sour cream (light)
		Yogurt (low-fat with
		    sugar)
			Buttermilk
			Cottage/cream cheese
			    or sour cream (1% or
			    fat-free)
			Extra-low-fat cheese
			Fruit yogurt (fat-free
			    with sweetener)
			Milk (skim)
			Soy milk (plain, low-fat)

CARBOHYDRATES

Cereals	All cold cereals except those listed as yellow- or green-light Granola Muesli (commercial)	Kashi Good Friends Shredded Wheat Bran	All-Bran Bran Buds Fibre First Kashi Go Lean Kashi Go Lean Crunch Oat Bran Porridge (old-fashioned rolled oats) Red River
Breads/Grains	Bagels Baguette Cookies Doughnuts Muffins Pancakes/Waffles White bread	Crispbreads (with fibre)* Whole-grain breads*	Crispbreads (high fibre, e.g., Wasa Fibre)* Green-light muffins (see pp. 257, 259) Whole-grain, high-fibre breads (min. 3g fibre per slice)*
Fruits (Fresh/Frozen)	Applesauce containing sugar Canned fruit in syrup Melons Most dried fruit	Apricots (fresh and dried)** Bananas Fruit cocktail in juice Kiwi Mango Papaya Pineapple	Apples Berries Cherries Grapefruit Grapes Oranges Peaches
Juices	Fruit drinks Prune Sweetened juices Watermelon	Apple (unsweetened) Grapefruit (unsweetened) Orange (unsweetened) Pear (unsweetened)	Eat the fruit rather than drink its juice
Vegetables	French fries Hash browns		Most vegetables

FATS

	Butter Hard margarine Peanut butter (regular and light) Tropical oils Vegetable shortening	Most nuts Natural nut butters Peanut butter (100% peanuts) Soft margarine (non-hydrogenated) Vegetable oils	Almonds* Canola oil* Hazelnuts* Olive oil* Soft margarine (non-hydrogenated, light)*

* Limit serving size (see page 25).
** For baking, it is acceptable to use a modest amount of dried apricots or cranberries.

Coffee and Tea

OK, this is a tough one. The trouble with coffee is caffeine. It's not a health problem in itself, but it does stimulate blood sugar levels. So in Phase I, try to cut out caffeine altogether. As unpleasant as it may be, caffeine withdrawal will end in a day or two. Cut down gradually: go from a medium coffee to a small; then try a half-caffeinated, half-decaf blend. Then limit yourself to decaffeinated coffee—some brands taste as good as the real thing.

Even better, switch to tea. It has only about one-third of the caffeine that coffee has, and black tea and green tea have health benefits as well: they're rich in antioxidants, and beneficial for heart health and reducing the risk of dementia. Green tea is also considered an anti-carcinogen. (My ninety-nine-year-old mother and her tea-drinking cronies are living proof!) Herbal teas, such as peppermint, chamomile and other blends, are fine too, as long as they contain no caffeine.

If no coffee is going to be a deal breaker, then go ahead, have one cup a day—but not a double espresso. If you take milk and sugar, make it skim milk and a sweetener such as Splenda.

Cereals

Another toughie. Most cold cereals contain hidden or not-so-hidden sugars, and are therefore red-light. Green-light cereals are high in fibre and/or protein; they have at least 10 grams per serving. All right, they're not a lot of fun by themselves, but you can liven them up with fresh, canned or frozen fruits, a few nuts and some fruit yogurt (fat-free, with sweetener).

My personal favourite cereal is good-old-fashioned oatmeal—not the instant type that comes in packets but the large-flake, slow-cooking kind. (They're starting to serve it in the smartest hotels now.) Large-flake oatmeal is not only low–G.I., but also low-calorie and has been shown to lower cholesterol. Yes, you have to cook it, but it takes only about three minutes or so in the microwave, and not much longer for one portion on the stovetop. Dress it up with fat-free fruit yogurt, sliced almonds, berries or unsweetened applesauce. It's also just fine with nothing but milk on it.

I probably receive more e-mails about people's delight at rediscovering oatmeal than about any other food or meal. Give it a try.

Juice

Always eat the fruit or vegetable rather than drink its juice. The fruit contains more fibre and nutrients than just its juice. This is particularly the case with commercially prepared juices. Also, as juice is a processed product, it has a higher G.I. because it is more rapidly digested than the parent fruit. Finally, a glass of juice has two and a half times the calories of a whole fresh orange.

Toast

Go ahead, but have no more than one slice per meal. Make sure your bread has at least 3 grams of fibre per slice. (Note: Some bread labels quote a two-slice serving, which should equal 6 grams per serving.) The best choice is 100% percent whole wheat or whole grain bread. White bread, cracked wheat or anything else made with white flour is red-light.

Butter and Jams

Butter is out. It's very high in saturated fat, and despite the protestations of the dairy industry, it's not good for your health or waistline. Yes, it does make things taste good—that's what fat does best. But you can still enjoy any one of a variety of light non-hydrogenated soft margarines, if you use only a teaspoon or so.

When buying fruit spreads, look for the "extra fruit/no sugar added" varieties. Fruit, not sugar, should be the first ingredient listed. These varieties taste great and don't have the calories of the usual commercial jams. Although I rarely plug brands, President's Choice Blue Menu jams are a good buy.

Dairy

Low-fat dairy products are an ideal green-light choice and an excellent source of protein. I have a glass of skim milk every morning. I admit that skim didn't taste great at first, but I weaned myself off 2 percent by switching to 1 percent before moving on to skim. Now 2 percent tastes like cream!

Fat-free yogurt with sugar substitute instead of sugar is ideal for breakfast, dessert or a snack, either by itself or added to fruits or cereals. Low-fat cottage cheese is also a top-rated green-light source of protein. Or you can make a low-fat soft cheese spread by letting yogurt drain in cheesecloth overnight in the refrigerator.

Regular full-fat dairy products, including whole milk and cream, cheese and butter, are loaded with saturated fat and should be avoided completely.

Eggs

Use liquid eggs, such as Naturegg Break Free or Omega Pro. They are lower in saturated fat and cholesterol than regular eggs, and they make wonderful omelettes. Otherwise, use egg whites. If you're eating a hotel breakfast, in most cases the kitchen is happy to make omelettes with egg whites only.

Bacon

Bacon is red-light because of its high saturated-fat content. However, there are tasty green-light alternatives—such as Canadian back bacon, and lean ham—that make great BLTs.

LUNCH

Lunch is usually the most problematic meal for my readers because they tend to eat it outside the home and in a hurry. Bringing your lunch to work is the easiest way to ensure you eat green-light. And there are other advantages to brown-bagging it, besides avoiding the temptation of a red-light lunch: it's cheaper, and it gives you downtime at your desk to read or catch up on paperwork. However, it's a good idea to actually get away from your desk altogether so you can be more mindful of what you are eating—rather than trying to work and eat at the same time. If you can get away from your desk for half an hour or so, try taking your lunch outside and adding a little exercise to your day. Here are the ground rules for making that brown bag a green-light bag. For a complete list of foods, see the Complete G.I. Diet Food Guide on pages 271–277.

PROTEIN			
Meat, Poultry, Fish, Eggs and Meat Substitutes	Ground beef (more than 10% fat)	Ground beef (lean)	All fish and seafood, fresh, frozen (no batter or breading) or canned (in water)
	Hamburgers	Lamb (lean cuts)	Beef (lean cuts)
	Hot dogs	Pork (lean cuts)	Chicken/Turkey breast (skinless)
	Pâté	Tofu	Egg whites
	Processed meats	Turkey bacon	Ground beef (extra-lean)
	Regular bacon	Whole regular eggs (preferably omega-3)	Lean deli ham
	Sausages		Liquid eggs (e.g., Break-Free)
			Tofu (soft)
			Veal

CARBOHYDRATES

| Breads/Grains | Bagels
Baguette/Croissants
Croutons
Cake/Cookies
Hamburger/Hot dog buns
Macaroni and cheese
Muffins/Doughnuts
Noodles (canned or
   instant)
Pancakes/Waffles
Pasta filled with cheese
   or meat
Pizza
Rice (short-grain, white,
   instant) | Crispbreads (with fibre,
   e.g., Ryvita High
   Fibre)
Pita (whole wheat)
Tortillas (whole wheat)
Whole-grain breads* | Crispbreads (high fibre,
   e.g., Wasa Fibre)*
Pasta (fettuccine,
   spaghetti, penne,
   vermicelli, linguine,
   macaroni)*
Pita (high fibre)
Quinoa
Rice (basmati, wild,
   brown, long-grain)*
Whole-grain, high-fibre
   breads (min. 3g fibre
   per slice)* |
| Fruits/Vegetables
(Fresh/Frozen) | Broad beans
French fries
Melons
Most dried fruit
Parsnips
Potatoes (mashed or
   baked)
Rutabaga | Apricots (fresh and
   dried)**
Artichokes
Bananas
Beets
Corn
Kiwi
Mango
Papaya
Pineapple
Potatoes (boiled)
Squash
Sweet potatoes
Yams | Apples
Arugula
Asparagus
Avocado*
Beans (green/wax)
Bell peppers
Blackberries
Blueberries
Broccoli
Brussels sprouts
Cabbage
Carrots
Cauliflower
Celery
Cherries
Cucumbers
Eggplant
Grapefruit
Grapes
Leeks
Lemons
Lettuce
Mushrooms
Olives*
Onions
Oranges (all varieties)
Peaches
Pears
Peas
Peppers (hot)
Pickles
Plums |

* Limit serving size (see page 25).
** For baking, it is acceptable to use a modest amount of dried apricots or cranberries.

Fruits/Vegetables (Fresh/Frozen)			Potatoes (new or small) Radishes Raspberries Snow peas Spinach Strawberries Tomatoes Zucchini
FATS			
	Butter Hard margarine Mayonnaise Peanut butter (regular, light) Salad dressings (regular) Tropical oils	Mayonnaise (light) Most nuts Peanut butter (100% peanuts) Salad dressings (light) Soft margarine (non-hydrogenated)	Almonds* Canola oil* Mayonnaise (fat-free) Olive oil* Salad dressings (low-fat, low-sugar) Soft margarine (non-hydrogenated, light)*
SOUPS			
	All cream-based soups Canned black bean Canned green pea Canned puréed vegetable Canned split pea	Canned chicken noodle Canned lentil Canned tomato	Chunky bean and vegetable soups (e.g., Campbell's Healthy Request, Healthy Choice) Homemade soups with green-light ingredients

* Limit serving size (see page 25).

Sandwiches

Sandwiches are a lunchtime staple, and it's no wonder: they're portable and easy to make, and they offer endless variety. They can also be a dietary disaster, but if you follow the suggestions below, you can keep your sandwiches green-light.

• Always use 100 percent whole wheat or high-fibre whole-grain bread (min. 3 grams of fibre per slice).

• Sandwiches should be served open-faced. Either pack components separately and assemble just before eating or make your sandwich with a "lettuce lining" that helps keep the bread from getting soggy.

• Include at least three vegetables, such as lettuce, tomato, red or green bell pepper, cucumber, sprouts or onion.

• Instead of spreading the bread with butter or margarine, use mustard or hummus.

• Add up to 4 ounces of cooked lean meat or fish: roast beef, turkey, shrimp or salmon.

• If you make tuna or chicken salad, use low-fat mayonnaise or low-fat salad dressing and celery.

• Mix canned salmon with malt vinegar or fresh lemon.

Salads

Preparing salads may seem more labour intensive than making sandwiches, but it doesn't have to be. Invest in a variety of reusable plastic containers so you can bring individual-sized salads to work. Keep a supply of green-light vinaigrette on hand, and wash greens ahead of time and store in paper towels in plastic bags. You'll find that salads are a creative way to use up leftovers with a minimum of fuss.

DINNER

Dinner is traditionally the main meal of the day, and the one where we may have a tendency to overeat. We usually have more time for eating at the end of the day, and we generally feel fatigued as well, which encourages us to consume more. But since we will probably be spending the evening relaxing before going to bed, rather than being active, it is important that we don't overdo it. For a complete list of foods, see the Complete G.I. Diet Food Guide on pages 271-277.

PROTEIN			
Meat, Poultry, Fish, Eggs and Meat Substitutes	Breaded fish and seafood Ground beef (more than 10% fat) Hamburgers Hot dogs Processed meats Sausages Sushi	Fish canned in oil Ground beef (lean) Lamb (lean cuts) Pork (lean cuts) Whole regular eggs (preferably omega-3)	All fish and seafood, fresh, frozen (not breaded or canned in oil) Beef (lean cuts) Chicken/Turkey breast (skinless) Egg whites Ground beef (extra-lean) Lean deli ham Liquid eggs (e.g., Break Free) Pork tenderloin Textured vegetable protein (TVP) Tofu (soft) Veal

DAIRY

Almond milk	Cheese (low-fat)	Buttermilk
Cheese	Cream cheese (light)	Cottage cheese (1% or fat-free)
Chocolate milk	Ice cream (low-fat)	Cream cheese (fat-free)
Coconut milk	Milk (1%)	Extra-low-fat cheese (e.g., Laughing Cow Light, Boursin Light)
Cottage cheese (whole or 2%)	Sour cream (light)	Frozen yogurt 1/2 cup, low-fat)
Evaporated millk	Yogurt (low-fat, with sugar)	Flavoured yogurt (non-fat with sweetener)
Goat milk		Ice cream (1/2 cup, low-fat and no added sugar)
Ice cream		Milk (skim)
Milk (whole or 2%)		Sour Cream (1% or less)
Rice milk		Soy milk (plain, low-fat)
Sour cream		Whey protein powder
Yogurt (whole or 2%)		

CARBOHYDRATES

Breads/Grains	Bagels	Pita (whole wheat)	Pasta (fettuccine, spaghetti, penne, vermicelli, linguine, macaroni)*
	Baguette/Croissants	Whole-grain breads*	Quinoa
	Cake/Cookies		Rice (basmati, wild, brown, long-grain)*
	Macaroni and cheese		Whole-grain, high-fibre breads (min. 3g fibre per slice)*
	Muffins/Doughnuts		
	Noodles (canned or instant)		
	Pasta filled with cheese or meat		
	Pizza		
	Rice (short-grain, white, instant)		
	Tortillas		
Fruits/Vegetables (Fresh/Frozen)	Broad beans	Apricots	Apples
	French fries	Bananas	Arugula
	Melons	Beets	Asparagus
	Most dried fruit	Corn	Avocado*
	Parsnips	Kiwi	Beans (green/wax)
	Potatoes (mashed or baked)	Mango	Bell peppers
		Papaya	Blackberries
		Pineapple	Blueberries
		Potatoes (boiled)	Broccoli
		Squash	Brussels sprouts
		Sweet potatoes	Cabbage
		Yams	Carrots
			Cauliflower
			Celery
			Cherries
			Cucumbers

* Limit serving size (see page 25).

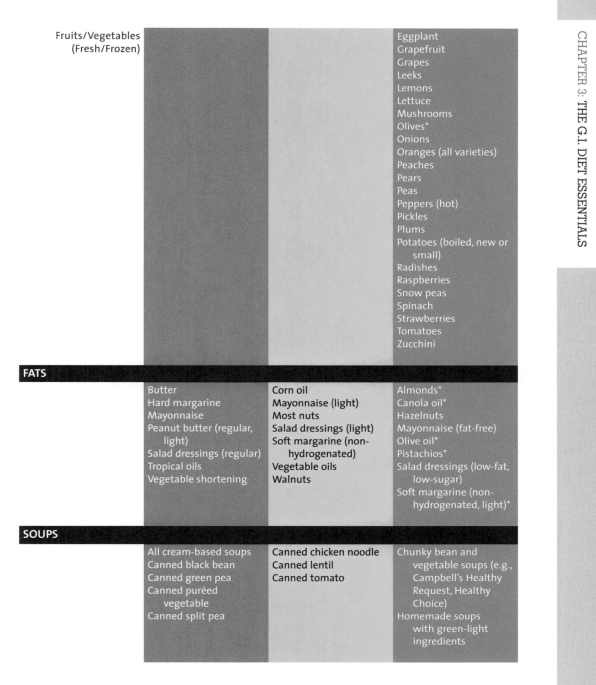

Fruits/Vegetables (Fresh/Frozen)		Eggplant
		Grapefruit
		Grapes
		Leeks
		Lemons
		Lettuce
		Mushrooms
		Olives*
		Onions
		Oranges (all varieties)
		Peaches
		Pears
		Peas
		Peppers (hot)
		Pickles
		Plums
		Potatoes (boiled, new or small)
		Radishes
		Raspberries
		Snow peas
		Spinach
		Strawberries
		Tomatoes
		Zucchini

FATS

Butter	Corn oil	Almonds*
Hard margarine	Mayonnaise (light)	Canola oil*
Mayonnaise	Most nuts	Hazelnuts
Peanut butter (regular, light)	Salad dressings (light)	Mayonnaise (fat-free)
Salad dressings (regular)	Soft margarine (non-hydrogenated)	Olive oil*
Tropical oils	Vegetable oils	Pistachios*
Vegetable shortening	Walnuts	Salad dressings (low-fat, low-sugar)
		Soft margarine (non-hydrogenated, light)*

SOUPS

All cream-based soups	Canned chicken noodle	Chunky bean and vegetable soups (e.g., Campbell's Healthy Request, Healthy Choice)
Canned black bean	Canned lentil	
Canned green pea	Canned tomato	
Canned puréed vegetable		Homemade soups with green-light ingredients
Canned split pea		

* Limit serving size (see page 25).

Protein

No dinner is complete without protein. Whether it is in the form of meat, poultry, seafood, beans or tofu, it should cover no more than one-quarter of your plate. A serving size should be 4 ounces,* which is roughly the size of the palm of your hand.

Red Meat

Though most red meat does contain saturated fat, there are ways to minimize it:

- Buy only low-fat meats such as top round beef. For hamburgers or spaghetti sauces, buy extra-lean ground beef. Veal and pork tenderloin are low in fat, too. As for juicy steaks, well, they are juicy because of the fat in them, so they're not a good choice.
- Trim any visible fat from the meat. Even a quarter inch of fat can double the total amount of fat in the meat.
- Broiling or grilling allows the excess fat from the meat to drain off. (Try one of those George Foreman–style fat-draining electric grills.)
- For stovetop cooking, use a non-stick pan with a little vegetable oil spray rather than oil. The spray goes further.

Poultry

Skinless chicken and turkey breast are excellent green-light choices. In the yellow-light category are skinless thighs, wings and legs, which are higher in fat.

Seafood

This is always a good green-light choice. Although certain cold-water fish, such as salmon and cod, have a relatively high oil content, this oil is omega-3 and is beneficial to your heart health. Shrimp and squid are fine, too, as long as they aren't breaded or battered. Fish and chips, alas, is out.

Beans (Legumes)

If you don't think you're into beans, it's time to re-evaluate! Beans are such an excellent source of so many good things: fibre, low-fat protein and "good" carbs that deliver nutrients while taking their time going through the digestive system. And they are a snap to incorporate into salads and soups to up the protein quotient. Chickpeas, lentils, navy beans, black beans, kidney beans—there's a bean for every day of the week. But watch out for canned pork and beans, which is high in sugar and fat, and avoid canned bean soups, which are processed to the point where their overall G.I. rating is too high. Homemade bean soups, however, are an excellent choice.

You will find several delicious recipes using beans in the recipes section of this book.

Tofu

You don't have to be a vegetarian to enjoy tofu, which is low in saturated fat and an excellent source of protein. While tofu is not necessarily a thriller on its own, it takes on the flavours of whatever seasonings and sauces it is cooked with. Seasoned tofu scrambles, for instance, are a good substitute for scrambled eggs. Choose soft tofu, which has up to one-third less fat than the firm variety.

Textured Vegetable Protein (TVP)

This is not a new device for pre-recording TV shows! TVP is a soy alternative to meat that looks a lot like ground beef, and can be used in the same ways—in lasagna, chili, stir-fries and spaghetti sauce. It's quite tasty and delivers the texture of meat. Our middle son, a vegetarian who has since left the nest, put us on to this versatile product.

Potatoes, Pasta, Rice

These carbohydrates should cover only one-quarter of the plate. Remember, with potatoes your first choice is boiled small or new potatoes. Most other choices, especially baked potatoes or french fries, are red-light. Sweet potatoes are a good lower–G.I. food, but since they tend to come in larger sizes, I suggest you save them for Phase II.

Your serving of pasta should be no more than $\frac{3}{4}$ cup cooked*—just until al dente. If you have rice, make it $\frac{2}{3}$ cup cooked basmati, wild, brown or long-grain rice.

Vegetables

Here you can put the measuring cup away. Eat as many vegetables and as much salad as you like; they should be the backbone of your meal. Always include at least two vegetables, and remember to cook them just until tender-crisp. Experiment with something you've never had before. Baby bok choy is delicious grilled, and rapini, a dark green vegetable that looks like broccoli with more leaves, is a nice change. The dark, curly green vegetables such as kale are full of good things, including folic acid.

* For Preliminary Phase servings see p. 25

Greens such as mesclun or baby spinach come conveniently pre-washed in bags. Frozen bags of mixed vegetables are also convenient and inexpensive; you can even toss the veggies into a saucepan, add tomato juice with a dollop of salsa and you have a quick vegetable soup.

DESSERT

Yes, dessert is part of the G.I. Diet—at least, the kind of dessert that is green-light and good for you. This includes most fruits, and low-fat dairy products, such as yogurt and ice cream sweetened with sugar substitute rather than sugar. You can also try silken or dessert tofu but watch the serving size (maximum of ½ cup). All my books have recipes for delicious green-light desserts.

SNACKS

Keep your digestive system busy and your energy up with between-meal snacks—four a day during the Preliminary Phase and three a day during Phase I.

Try to eat balanced snacks that include a bit of protein and carbohydrates; for example, a piece of fruit with a few nuts, or cottage cheese with celery sticks.

A convenient snack for when you're on the go is half a nutrition bar. Be careful when choosing one: most are full of cereal and sugar. The ones to look for have 12 to 15 grams of protein per 50g bar. Balance and ZonePerfect bars are two examples. Shopper's Drug Mart's Life Brand Sportzone Energy Bar is a best buy.

Keep in mind that many snacks and desserts labelled "low-fat" or "sugar-free" aren't necessarily green-light. Sugar-free instant puddings and "low-fat" muffins are still high–G.I. because they contain highly processed grains.

SNACKS		
Bagels	Bananas	Almonds*
Candy	Dark chocolate (70%	Applesauce
Cookies	cocoa)	(unsweetened)
Crackers	Ice cream (low-fat)	Canned peaches/pears in
Doughnuts	Most nuts	juice or water
Flavoured gelatin (all	Popcorn (light,	Cottage cheese (1% or
varieties)	microwavable)	fat-free)
French fries		Extra-low-fat cheese
Ice cream		(e.g., Laughing Cow
Muffins (commercial)		Light, Boursin Light)
Popcorn (regular)		Frozen yogurt (low-fat)

* Limit serving size (see page 25).

SNACKS

Potato chips		Fruit yogurt (fat-free
Pretzels		with sweetener)
Pudding		Hazelnuts*
Raisins		Homemade green-light
Rice cakes		snacks (see pages
Sorbet		256)
Tortilla chips		Ice cream (low-fat and
Trail mix		no added sugar)
White bread		Most fresh/frozen fruit
		Most fresh/frozen
		vegetables
		Nutrition bars**
		Pickles
		Pumpkin seeds
		Sugar-free hard candies
		Sunflower seeds

** 180–225 calorie bars, e.g., ZonePerfect or Balance Bars

WHAT DO I DRINK?

Because liquids don't trip our satiety mechanisms, it's a waste to take in calories through them. Also, many beverages are high in calories. Juice, for example, is a processed product, and has a much higher G.I. than the fruit or vegetable it is made from. A glass of orange juice contains nearly two and a half times the calories of a fresh orange! So eat the fruit or vegetable rather than drink its juice. That way you'll get all the benefits of its nutrients and fibre while consuming fewer calories.

As well, stay away from any beverage that contains added sugar or caffeine. As I explained earlier, caffeine stimulates blood sugar levels. So no coffee or soft drinks containing caffeine in Phase I.

That said, fluids are an important part of any diet (I'm sure you're all familiar with the eight-glasses-a-day prescription). The following are your best green-light choices:

Water

The cheapest, easiest and best thing to drink is plain water. Seventy percent of our body consists of water, which is needed for digestion, circulation, regulation of body temperature, lubrication of joints and healthy skin. We can live for months without food, but we can survive only a few days without water.

Don't feel you have to drink eight glasses of water a day in addition to other beverages. Milk, tea and soft drinks all contribute to the eight-glasses-a-day recommendation. But do try to drink a glass of water before each meal—it will help you feel fuller so that you don't overeat. Add a slice of lemon or lime for flavour if you dislike plain water.

Skim Milk

After a skeptical start, I've grown to really enjoy skim milk, and I like to drink it with breakfast and lunch, which tend to be a little short on protein. Skim milk is an ideal green-light food.

Soft Drinks

If you're used to drinking soft drinks, you can still enjoy the sugar- and caffeine-free diet ones. People often treat regular soft drinks and fruit juices as nonfoods, but this is how extra calories slip by us.

Tea

Although black and green teas do contain caffeine, the amount is only about one-third of that of coffee. Tea has health benefits as well. Black and green teas contain antioxidant properties that help protect against heart disease and Alzheimer's. In fact, tea has more flavonoids (antioxidants) than any vegetable tested. Two cups of black or green tea have the same amount of antioxidants as 7 cups of orange juice or 28 cups of apple juice.

So tea in moderation is fine—minus the sugar and cream, of course. Try some new varieties: Darjeeling, Earl Grey, English Breakfast or spicy chai (with sugar substitute). Herbal teas, as long as they are caffeine-free, are also a green-light option, though they lack the flavonoids. Iced tea is acceptable if it's sugar-free.

Alcohol

Alcohol is generally a disaster for any weight-loss program. It puts your blood sugar on a roller coaster: you go up and feel great, then come down and feel like having another drink, or eating the whole bowl of peanuts. Alcohol also contains a lot of calories. So in Phase I, put away the corkscrew and the ice cube tray.

Now that you know how the G.I. Diet works, it's time to get ready to start. In the next chapter, I'll outline the steps for launching you into the program.

TO SUM UP

- In the Preliminary Phase and Phase I, eat only green-light foods.
- Eat three balanced meals plus four snacks a day in the Preliminary Phase and three balanced meals plus three snacks a day in Phase I.
- Pay attention to portion size: palm of your hand for protein, and a quarter plate for pasta, potatoes or rice. Use common sense and eat moderate amounts.
- Drink plenty of fluids, including an 8-ounce glass of water with meals and snacks (but no caffeine or alcohol).

Chapter Four
Before You Start

The G.I. Diet it not so much a diet as a completely new and permanent way of eating. This is without question the most important message in this book and particularly relevant to diabetes. Unfortunately, most people view diets as a short-term change in eating habits that are ditched once weight-loss targets have been achieved. They then revert to their old dietary habits and, not suprisingly, they are soon back at their original weight, or worse.

The G.I. Diet is the way you will eat for the rest of your life. The one constant refrain I've received from the tens of thousands of successful readers is that this is a new way of eating that has become a permanent part of their lives.

Your motivation to lose weight is high, and with the G.I. Diet you now have the action plan that will help you make those unwanted pounds disappear. Still, to be successful you will have to make some significant changes in your life, and the better prepared you are, the better equipped you will be to handle any challenges that may arise. The following six steps will get you off to the best possible start.

1. GO SEE YOUR DOCTOR.

Before starting any major change in your eating patterns, check with your doctor to see if you have any concerns that could affect your weight-loss plans. As you lose weight, your health will certainly improve, and it will be wonderfully motivating to learn that your blood glucose levels have improved or that your blood pressure has gone down. It may even be possible to change or reduce any medications you might be taking.

2. ASSESS WHETHER IT'S THE RIGHT TIME TO START.

Are you in the middle of a job change? A major house renovation or move? Is it the week before Christmas or before the cruise you've been planning for a year? Then it's probably not the best time to start a new way of eating. Some life events will make it harder—or even impossible—for you to give the program the attention it needs or to stick with it. Choose a period when your life is relatively stable and when you have time to learn new eating habits—not when your stress levels are even higher than usual. If your enthusiasm for a new slim and healthier you is high and the timing is right, then there's no better moment than the present!

3. SET YOUR WEIGHT-LOSS TARGET.

It's important to have a healthy, realistic weight-loss target in mind before starting the program. A good place to start is the BMI table on pages 26–27, not the glossy pages of a fashion or fitness magazine. Being too thin or too heavy is not good. Your health is at risk if your BMI is below 18.5 or above 25. Remember, the BMI table is only a guide.

The other measurement you should concern yourself with is your waist measurement, which is an even better predictor of the state of your health than your weight. Abdominal fat is more than just a weight problem. Recent research has shown that abdominal fat acts almost like a separate organ in the body, except this "organ" is a destructive one that releases harmful proteins and free fatty acids, increasing your risk of life-threatening conditions, especially diabetes and heart disease.

If you are female and have a waist measurement of 35 inches or more, or are male with a waist measurement of over 37 inches, you are at risk of endangering your health. Women with a measurement of 37 inches or more, and men with a measurement over 40 inches are at serious risk of heart disease, stroke, cancer and diabetes.

So I have your attention now! Make sure that you measure correctly: put a tape measure around your waist just above navel level till it fits snugly, without cutting into your flesh. Do not adopt the walking-down-the-beach-sucking-in-your-stomach stance. Just stand naturally. There's no point in trying to fudge the numbers, because the only person you're kidding is yourself.

Now that you know your BMI and waist measurement, you can set your weight-loss target and know roughly how long it will take you to reach that goal. When you lose weight in a healthy way, you can expect to lose about one pound per week. I say "about" because most people do not lose weight at a fixed and steady rate. The usual pattern is to lose more at the start of the diet, when you are losing mostly water weight, followed by a series of drops and plateaus. The closer you get to your target weight, the slower your weight loss will be. If you are planning to lose up to 20 percent of your body weight—for example, if you weigh 150 pounds and want to lose 30 pounds—assume this will take you thirty weeks, one pound per week. If you have more than 20 percent to shed, the good news is that you will lose at a faster rate. This is simply because your larger body weight requires more calories just to keep operating than someone who is lighter. Still, be prepared for measured results—it took you a while to put on those extra pounds and it will take some time to lose them. Be patient and know that once that weight is gone, it will be gone forever as you keep it off in Phase II of the program.

Although I recommend recording your progress, please don't get obsessed with numbers on the scale. Many people find themselves losing inches before they register any weight loss. Clothes start feeling a little looser, and before you know it you are down a dress size or getting into your old jeans. Soon you'll probably have to buy new clothes. My readers often tell me I should have warned them about the extra cost of refurbishing their closet!

4. GIVE YOUR KITCHEN A GREEN-LIGHT MAKEOVER.

Take a look in your fridge—what do you see? Two jars of mayonnaise, some leftover cheddar and a lot of sugar-laden condiments in jars? Now open the cupboards: what's the cookie and cracker situation? Now is the time to do an honest evaluation of what you tend to keep on hand. Consult the Complete G.I. Diet Food Guide (pages 271–277) and throw out anything that's in the red-light column. Be ruthless. If you always have chips on hand, you will eat them. If you keep Goldfish crackers around "for the kids," you can be sure that they won't be the only ones snacking on them. Give the unopened food items and cans to your skinny neighbours or local food bank.

5. EAT BEFORE YOU SHOP.

You know what happens when you drop by the supermarket on your way home from work, famished—before you know it you've bought the biggest tray of cannelloni ever made. The worst mistake you can make is to go shopping on an empty stomach. You'll only be tempted to fill your cart with high–G.I., calorie-rich foods.

6. SHOP GREEN-LIGHT.

For those of you who prefer a day-by-day guide to your planning, for each week of the G.I. Diet Diabetes Clinic in Part II, I provide a complete meal and snack plan and a grocery list. If you'd rather not follow the plan, go back and consult Chapter 3 to get some ideas of what you'd like to have for breakfast, lunch, dinner and snacks during your first week on the G.I. Diet; have a look at the Complete G.I. Diet Food Guide on pages 271–277; and peruse the recipe section of this book, or any of my other books, such as the *G.I. Diet Cookbook*. Write a shopping list and head out to the supermarket. Your first few green-light shopping trips will require a bit more time and attention than usual, as you familiarize yourself with green-light eating and meal planning. But don't worry: before long your new shopping and eating habits will become second nature.

Since it would be impossible to include every brand available in today's enormous supermarkets in the Complete G.I. Diet Food Guide, I've listed categories of food rather than individual brands, except in cases where clarification is needed, or where there is an especially useful product available. This means that you will have to pay some attention to food labels when comparing brands.

HOW TO READ A FOOD LABEL

When reading a food label, there are six factors to consider when making the best green-light choice:

1. SERVING SIZE

Is the serving size realistic, or has the manufacturer lowered it to make the calories and fat levels look better than the competition's? When comparing brands, ensure that you are comparing the same serving size.

2. CALORIES

The brand with the least amount of calories is obviously the best choice. Some brands flagged as "low-fat" still have plenty of calories, so don't be fooled by the diet-friendly slogans. Calories are calories, whether they come from fat or sugar.

3. FAT

Look at the amount of fat, which is often expressed as a percentage, say 2 percent (good) or 20 percent (forget it). Then check to see what sort of fat it is. You want foods that are low-fat, with minimal or no saturated fats and trans fats. Remember that trans fats are often called "hydrogenated oils" or "partially hydrogenated oils."

4. FIBRE

Foods with lots of fibre have a low G.I., so this is an important component. When comparing brands, choose the one with higher fibre.

5. SUGAR

Choose brands that are low in sugar. Again, watch for brands advertised as "low-fat." Companies will sometimes quietly bump up the sugar content to make up for any perceived loss of taste. This often happens with yogurts and cereals.

Sugars are sometimes listed as dextrose, glucose, fructose or sucrose; regardless of the form, it's sugar. For information on sugar substitutes such as sugar alcohols, agave nectar and stevia, see page 66.

6. SODIUM

Sodium (salt) increases water retention, which doesn't help when you are trying to lose weight. It also contributes to premenstrual bloating in women and is a factor in hypertension (high blood pressure). Diabetics are at particular risk of high blood pressure. Combine it with excess weight and you move up to the front of the risk line for heart disease and stroke. Low-sodium products are therefore preferable.

The Recommended Dietary Allowance (RDA) for sodium is 2,500 mg, but this is generally regarded as too high. The U.S. National Academy of Science's new recommendation of 1,500 mg makes more sense. Since the average North American consumption of sodium per person per day is over 3,000 mg, it goes without saying that most of us could stand to cut back. However, if you have a BMI over 30 and have any blood pressure, circulation or heart problems, you need to be even more vigilant about seeking out low-sodium brands. Canned foods such as soups are often very high in sodium, as are many fast foods and processed foods.

You've talked to your doctor, decided there's no better time than the present to lose weight and get healthy, set your weight-loss target, cleared your kitchen of fat-building foods and restocked your pantry with delicious green-light choices. Now all you have to do is eat green-light meals and snacks each day and you're well on your way to your new trim self. In the next section, you'll find a week-by-week guide to all the challenges and issues that will come up as you follow the G.I. Diet for the first thirteen weeks. By the end of it you will know everything there is to know to achieve your weight-loss dreams, and you'll have lost a significant amount of weight, lowered your blood sugar levels along the way and maybe even reduced your diabetes medications.

TO SUM UP

The six steps to get you launched into the G.I. Diet are:

- Go see your doctor.
- Assess whether it's the right time to start.
- Set you weight-loss target.
- Give your kitchen a green-light makeover.
- Eat before you shop.
- Shop green-light.

PART II: The G.I. Diet Diabetes Clinic

Week 1
Getting Started

Welcome to the G.I. Diet Diabetes Clinic. You are starting out on one of the biggest and most important adventures of your life. This is a journey that is truly life changing as you will have the opportunity to reduce your weight, your blood sugar levels and perhaps even your diabetes medications.

Please note that this book is not a primer on diabetes or pre-diabetes. There are many excellent books on the subject as well as other resources that are available through the American and Canadian Diabetes Associations. If you require medical advice, please ask your health care provider.

TARGET WEIGHT

The first thing I would like you to do is fill in your current measurements below as well as your target weight, so that you have a baseline with which to compare your progress and a place to remind yourself of your ultimate weight-loss goal. There is nothing more motivating than recording your success, so I will be asking you to write down your weight and waist measurements at the end of each week. Be sure to measure yourself at the same time of the day each week since a meal or even a bowel movement can make a difference of a pound or two at a time when every pound counts! An ideal time is first thing in the morning, before breakfast.

Talking of scales, it is important that you are able to have an accurate measure of your weight. Many of you are probably using scales you have had around for years. Chances are they are the analogue type (either with a pointer or a rotating disk). Over time, the springs in these types of scales stretch and become wildly inaccurate. Do yourself a favour and purchase a digital scale. They can be bought for well under $50.

Current Weight: _____

Current Waist: _____

Target Weight: _____

A few words about setting your weight target. The international standard for weight measurement is the Body Mass Index or BMI. Measure your BMI on the BMI table, pages 26–27. The ideal BMI range is 19–24. (For a more detailed rundown on where you might fit in this range, see Frame Size, page 22.)

However, it is important that you've set your goals. Everyone has different motivations for losing weight and neither I nor the BMI table can do this for you. So set your target weight goals and write them on the previous page.

Remember, you are starting on a journey. Don't expect miracles. The weight will come off.

For those with a BMI of over 30 who may feel overwhelmed by the task ahead, you do have one advantage over your skinnier compatriots in that you will lose weight at a faster rate.

You are starting on a new way of eating that will be your way of eating for the rest of your life. Congratulations for making the decision to take control. Enjoy the ride!

DIABETES AND WEIGHT

Eighty to 90 percent of Type II diabetes is caused by overweight and obesity. In simple terms, excess fat, especially around the abdomen, leads to the development of insulin resistance. Reducing your weight and inches substantially increases your chances of reversing the process and ultimately reducing your insulin resistance levels.

The glycemic index does double duty. It helps you not only stabilize your blood sugars but also lose weight. As low–G.I. foods digest more slowly, you remain feeling fuller for longer. In other words, they are more satiating. Therefore, you eat less, and eating less without going hungry is the key to permanent weight loss. It sounds so simple and it really is. In short, we will be helping you to deal with both the symptoms of the disease—your blood sugar levels—as well as the root cause of the disease itself—being overweight.

Unfortunately, we can gain weight as a result of age-related factors such as the following:

Hormones: In women, both estrogen and progesterone hormones become depleted during menopause, and this interferes with appetite control. Men experience a similar process known as andropause except that the hormone change is a reduction in testosterone.

Metabolism: This is the rate at which your body burns calories. As we age, our metabolic rate drops naturally. If you burn calories more slowly then you need fewer calories. And burning fewer calories without reducing your calorie input inevitably leads to weight gain.

Muscle mass: Muscles are the body's largest calorie consumers and we start losing muscle mass from the age of twenty. This muscle loss really accelerates during post-menopause—for men it's after sixty years—which means again you're burning fewer calories and therefore putting on the pounds if you haven't adjusted your calorie consumption.

Physical activity: As we approach our fifties, many of us become less active. Child rearing and its associated activity are largely over. Exercise becomes more of an effort and we become more conscious of the wear and tear on our bodies along with the inevitable aches and pains. Less exercise means fewer calories burned—and we know where the surplus calories are being stored!

Lifestyle: As many of us now have fewer family-raising responsibilities and are entering our peak earnings years, we tend to eat out and travel more. Eating out tends to be a calorie-rich experience. Calories taken in must equal calories expended or the surplus gets stored as fat.

The one common element in all the factors I've mentioned is calorie intake and expenditure. The two must be brought into balance—and that is what the G.I. Diet is all about. I will show you how to reduce your calorie intake painlessly and without going hungry or feeling deprived. The traffic-light coding means you never have to count calories or points, or weigh and measure your food. The G.I. Diet is a nutritious, balanced diet that will keep you healthy and reduce your risk of major diseases, including most cancers (including breast cancer), heart disease, stroke, dementia and, of course, diabetes. The evidence that food is the most important controllable risk factor in our health is overwhelming. While exercise is important for overall good health, it is a poor tool when it comes to losing weight. As you will read later, losing weight is 90 percent diet and 10 percent exercise. However, when you reach your target weight, exercise is essential to help you maintain that weight and improve your health.

At the age of 35, weighing 277 pounds and struggling with high blood pressure, I visited my doctor who decided it was time for a full-blown blood workup. The next week devastating news came to me: I was diagnosed with Type II diabetes, high cholesterol along with hypertension. I am no stranger to diabetes as my grandmother lost both of her legs to amputation and eventually died from this terrible disease. I thought I was doomed.

About a week later I stumbled across a small book called The G.I. Diet. *This book has become my Bible. I read it, followed it, and I am happy to tell you that I was thrilled when the weight started to come off. Five months later, my blood pressure was back to normal, my cholesterol was normal, and my glucose levels were that of a NON-diabetic. All my medications were stopped and I was monitored often to make sure I was maintaining healthy readings and still losing weight! I have lost 108 pounds in the year's time! No one can believe I have lost all this weight with no pills, no surgery, no "diet." I tell them all I am living the G.I. way. Not only have I lost and am still losing with hardly any effort, but also my husband has lost 40 pounds, and my now ten-year-old son has lost 10 pounds. Rick, I cannot tell you what this has done for me. I have been saved, given a new life, and a better outlook on my future with my family!*

Your biggest (well, skinnier) fan!
Jennifer

WHY DO YOU WANT TO LOSE WEIGHT?

Other than decreasing your insulin resistance, everyone has their own reasons for wanting to lose weight. Let's look at the most common reasons and see if they match yours.

BODY IMAGE

You want to look better. Weight loss boosts self-esteem and confidence for women in particular. It's amazing the difference the loss of just a few pounds can make, not only in how you look in your clothes but also in how you feel about yourself.

HEALTH

The single greatest risk to your health is your weight—as evidenced by the U.S. Surgeon General who identified obesity as that country's number-one health risk.

Excess weight is responsible for insulin resistance, which not only has an impact upon diabetics like you but also is linked directly to other major diseases such as hypertension—a harbinger of heart disease and stroke—as well as high cholesterol levels and many forms of cancer. The importance of reducing your weight, especially around your middle, is critical not only to your immediate diabetic health but also to your health in general.

ENERGY

Being overweight means you have more to carry around, which translates into flagging energy levels; sore back, hips and knees; and decreased mobility. The problem is that we don't realize what weight actually weighs. Take a shopping bag and fill it up with, say, 20 pounds of food cans/books (use bathroom scales) and carry it up and down two flights of stairs. You'll be glad to put the bag down. I have no idea how some people carry around 50 or more extra pounds all the time. I doubt if many of them could actually lift that weight!

Below, I would like you to write your personal top three reasons for wanting to lose weight. Take a moment to be clear about your reasons and be absolutely honest—this is for your eyes only. Later on, being able to come back to this page and read what you have written will go a long way toward keeping you motivated.

My Top Three Reasons for Losing Weight:

1. _____

_____

_____

2. _____

_____

_____

3. _____

_____

_____

MAKING PERMANENT CHANGE

As all of you know only too well, some 95 percent of diets fail and they fail for one simple reason: people just can't stay on them. Research has shown there are three principal reasons for this inability to stay with a diet:

1. You feel hungry or deprived.
2. It is too complex or time consuming, and you don't want to spend the rest of your life counting calories or points, or weighing and measuring foods.
3. You feel unhealthy and lack energy.

Well, on the G.I. Diet you will not go hungry or feel deprived. You will never have to count another calorie or point again—just follow the traffic lights. You will feel healthy and energetic eating the nutritious green-light way. This is not so much a diet as a new and permanent way of eating. No more yo-yo dieting. This is the way to lose weight permanently.

If there is only one thought I can leave with you in this first week, it is that if you wish to lose weight permanently, then you have to permanently change the way you eat.

It sounds simplistic but that is exactly why most diets and dieters fail time and time again. The assumption that you can go on a diet for a limited period of time and lose the weight you want to lose and then simply go back to your old way of eating will guarantee failure. Chances are that you will regain all the weight you have lost and perhaps even more.

Ultimately, the critical ingredient is you. I can provide you with the knowledge, tools and counsel to help make this an easy, simple and relatively painless transition to a new way of eating. But you have to make the commitment for it to work. Whether it's giving up smoking, getting fit or losing weight, nothing can be achieved until you decide you want to make it happen.

5 TOP TIPS

Here are my top five tips for helping you to achieve your weight-loss goals:

1. EAT THREE MEALS/THREE SNACKS PER DAY

Always eat three meals and three snacks per day. Breakfast is particularly important. The idea is to keep your tummy busy all day digesting green-light foods.

2. REMEMBER THE 90 PERCENT RULE

The G.I. Diet is not a straitjacket. Most people are successful if they stay with the diet 90 percent of the time. That additional 10 percent can be used for special treats: that unavoidable drink, or lunch out with the friends who love all the "wrong" foods.

3. DON'T RUSH YOUR MEALS

Eat slowly. Do not rush your meals as it can take half an hour for the brain to realize the stomach is full—a principal reason we overeat. Always put your fork down between mouthfuls.

4. EXERCISE

Initially, exercise is not that important as the change in diet will account for at least 90 percent of your weight loss. However, as you get closer to your target weight, exercise will become more important.

5. PORTIONS

Except for the dozen or so food items that have designated serving sizes, as listed on page 25, we leave green-light serving sizes primarily up to you. However, moderation is the key. Remember, the only person you are kidding is yourself.

E-CLINIC DIARIES

Each week I share some of the important questions or comments that the participants in the original diabetes e-clinic made in their weekly diaries that you might find helpful on the journey to your target weight. The first couple of weeks are always the most challenging as your body adapts to this new healthy way of eating. Changes in shopping, meals and eating patterns, along with your body's "hey, what's going on here" response, can all be a little unsettling at first. This will soon pass as you rapidly adapt to the green-light way of eating that will shortly become second nature.

Q: It is now day 3 of my journey and I'm finding it very difficult at certain times of the day. My mornings are great; I eat a bowl of steel-cut oats with a dash of maple syrup, a grapefruit, a small handful of raw almonds and a coffee plus a big glass of water and this takes me through to 11:30. Lunches are no problem because I love hearty soups (made with beans or some sort of protein) with a slice of grain bread, a couple of pieces of fruit, a glass of milk. At 3:00 to 4:00 I am ravenous!! And I get the same hunger pangs in the evening even though I have had a late-afternoon snack, a green-light dinner and a bedtime snack. I almost feel sick and headachey, definitely grumpy and depleted of energy. I suppose my body is adjusting, but being hungry is dominating my thoughts and my being. I have to admit I have huge cravings for something sugary. What can I do to keep the hunger pangs at bay? — Kate

A: This is not an unusual reaction during the first couple of weeks or so as your body adjusts to the new regime. I note that you are not including a mid-morning snack, which I strongly encourage. Also your lunch sounds a little thin on protein as you have to have a heck of a lot of beans in your soup in order to deliver a sufficient amount. Unless soups are prepared from scratch at home, virtually all commercially prepared soups are high–G.I. and therefore red-light. The problem is that commercial soups are processed at high temperatures to avoid spoilage, which almost doubles the G.I. rating versus a homemade soup. Change your lunches along the lines suggested in the book and you will avoid those mid-afternoon blues. That will give you more staying power and mean that you are not starving by dinnertime. That in turn will help you avoid hunger pangs later in the evening.

Q: What is non-hydrogenated margarine made from and why use something that is manufactured and not natural? I know that butter is saturated and I don't ever use much, but at least our bodies recognize it as a natural food. We have stayed away from anything hydrogenated for many years now and margarine has always been a real no-no because it is not natural. — Trish

A: Margarines are made principally from vegetable oils, which are high in the good oils (polyunsaturated and monounsaturated) and low in saturated.

A good soft non-hydrogenated margarine such as Becel consists of 80 percent vegetable oils (almost exclusively canola/sunflower oils) of which only 5 percent are saturated. This is about as "natural" as you can get. The rest is made up of whey protein, vitamins and stabilizers. Today's margarines are a lot different from earlier versions when concern for saturated fats was not on the health agenda. Much of the misinformation on margarine comes from the dairy industry that correctly saw margarine as a major threat to its butter monopoly.

Q: I am not quitting coffee. I am down to 2 cups a day and will become homicidal without it! Is it ok to continue? —Carol

A: There is increasing evidence that although coffee may have some beneficial impact on preventing diabetes, it certainly does not once you have been diagnosed. It's the caffeine in coffee that is the villain in that it increases blood sugar levels. There is an excellent update on this on WebMD.com (http://diabetes.webmd.com/news/20080128/caffeine-risks-may-rattle-diabetics).

There are some excellent decaffeinated coffees on the market. I've tried several at-home "tests" at dinner parties and no one could tell one from the other.

And for those of you who would like to experience a fast-forward, read the following "confession" from Michelle:

I wanted to tell you that I actually semi-started your diet 8 weeks ago . . . I had been on your e-mail list for years, but had never actually followed through with the G.I. diet, as I was so sure that this would be the same as all the other diets I've tried—a big disappointment, followed by a larger gain! . . . What I don't think I told you is that I started out eight weeks ago at 191.4 pounds!! I started slowly eliminating the things your book said I should—although I didn't go "gung ho" for the first few weeks, I still managed to lose 5 pounds right away, and have continued with a pound or two a week since then [current weight 177 pounds].

What I am the most excited about is the control over my blood sugars that has occurred with your diet. As I sit here in tears, literally, I have taken a fasting blood sugar reading of 6.6!!!! To understand how amazing that is, you'd have to know my history as a diabetic. When I was first diagnosed my blood sugar was a whopping 29.9. Within a few days of medication we had it down to the teens, and then to the single digits for my pre-lunch, pre-dinner, and bedtime readings, but never, in the 6 years that I've been diabetic have my fasting blood sugars . . . my first thing in the morning readings ever even been in the single digits . . . let alone at 6.6!!

You can't imagine how excited I was the first time I got a single-digit reading, after only 1 week of attempting your diet. That first week, I lost 5 pounds, and had a morning reading of 9.9. The readings since have only crept into the 10's once. The readings have steadily been declining—8.4, 7.7 and now this! My morning averages for the years preceding this had been at best 12.6, 11.8, 12.4.

I am so grateful already, and we've only just begun. I can't wait to get my next HBa1C—my doctor is going to be so happy, and hopefully she'll even cut down on some of my medications. So already, thank you, thank you, thank you. I'm excited to see how far we can go together and how much better control I can get!

Now, congratulate yourself for getting through the first week on the program, and record your measurements below. Also, take the time to write about your experiences and feelings this week. Diaries provide an opportunity to reflect on your progress, which helps reveal issues you might have to work on, ways of thinking that might be holding you back and strategies that could work well for you.

For Week 1, please see optional meal plan A on pages 173–174 in Part 4.

Week 1 Weight: _____

Week 1 Waist: _____

WEEK 1 DIARY

_____

_____

_____

_____

Week 2
Preparing Food
the Green-Light Way

At this point in the clinic, enthusiasm is usually at a high. However, it does take a week or two for your body to become accustomed to this new way of eating. Be aware that the numbers on the scale may not have changed much or at all yet. Keep the faith!

> *My husband was recently diagnosed with Type II diabetes. I went straight to the bookstore for answers. Loaded with information, I read and read. The information in most of the books on how to eat didn't seem right for people with blood sugar problems. We went to the education classes at our local hospital and were appalled by the information given to people with a chronic disease. Back at the bookstore, determined to help my husband, I ran across* The G.I. Diet. *This makes sense, I thought. The red, yellow and green categories are easy to use. Almost immediately his blood sugar was near normal. Four months later his A1C went from 11.4 to 6.1—from dangerous to near normal. The 44 pounds he's lost so far from our new diet is amazing. I wish the doctors we'd talked to were more informed about this not-so-new research. I am thankful to have read a book we can use for a lifetime—a long and healthy life . . .*
>
> *Thank you,*
> *Cathy*

Remember that our target weight loss is an *average* of one pound per week (see page 45). If you have a BMI of 33 or over, you may lose an average of up to two pounds per week especially in the first couple of months. It took you many years to achieve your current weight so don't fret if this seems a slow start. The G.I. Diet is not a quick-fix, so-called miracle diet. Instead it is a highly nutritious way of eating that will improve your health, lower you blood sugars and enable you to lose weight—and keep it off. Keep in mind what I said in Week 1: if you wish to lose weight permanently you must permanently change the way you eat.

TURNING YOUR STANDBYS INTO GREEN-LIGHT RECIPES

I'm going to have to be in the kitchen more [and] forced to get out of my cooking rut. I can no longer have the quick fix. Because I've been overweight forever, I think I have a mental block about baking and putting too much time into cooking . . . — Sheri

It's easy to make many of your own standby recipes green-light by following the guidelines below. You don't have to necessarily use the recipes listed in this book.

GREEN-LIGHT INGREDIENTS
First, ensure that all the ingredients in the recipe are green-light. If there are any red- or yellow-light ingredients, either omit or replace them with a green-light alternative. Some red- and yellow-light food can be used in recipes if there is a very limited quantity, such as $\frac{1}{2}$ cup of wine in a dish that will serve six people, or $\frac{1}{4}$ cup raisins in a salad for four. Full-flavoured cheeses can also occasionally be used sparingly. For example, a tablespoon or two of grated Parmesan cheese sprinkled over a casserole will add flavour without too many calories. As long as the red- and yellow-light ingredients are used in very limited quantities and not as a core ingredient, they will not have a significant impact on the overall G.I. or green-light rating of the recipe.

FIBRE
The fibre content of the recipe is critical. Fibre, both soluble and insoluble, is key to the overall G.I. rating of a recipe. The more, the better. If your recipe is light on fibre, consider adding fibre boosters such as oats, bran, whole grains or beans.

FAT
The recipes should be low in fat with little to no saturated fat. If fat is called for, use vegetable oil. Canola and olive oil are your best choices, but use as little as possible, as all fats are calorie-dense.

SUGAR

Never add sugar or sugar-based ingredients such as corn syrup or molasses. There are some excellent sugar substitutes on the market. My favourite is Splenda, or sucralose, which was developed from a sugar base but does not have as many calories. It works well in cooking and baking. Measure it by volume (not weight) to exactly replace sugar. For example, 1 tablespoon sugar = 1 tablespoon Splenda. Note that Brown Splenda is 50 percent sugar and is therefore not recommended. Sugar Twin Brown is an acceptable alternative.

Other sugar alternatives such as the sugar alcohols malitol and xylitol (all sugar alcohol names end in "tol") contain about 60 percent of the calories found in sugar. They do metabolize more slowly than sugar, which gives them a lower G.I. But as they are less sweet to the taste than sugar, manufacturers tend to use more, which defeats the whole purpose of using them to reduce calories. So though preferable to sugar, they carry an unnecessary calorie load and are therefore not recommended. Another sugar alternative is fructose, the sugar found in fruit. Though it has a lower G.I. than sugar, it still has the same number of calories and again is not recommended.

Two other natural sweeteners growing in popularity are agave nectar and stevia. Agave nectar contains fructose, which is low–G.I. and though sweeter than sugar contains the same number of calories. Stevia is an excellent alternative though some people, including me, don't like the aftertaste.

PROTEIN

Be sure that the recipe contains protein, or that you are serving it alongside some protein to round out the meal. Protein helps slow the digestive process, which effectively lowers the G.I. of a recipe. It is also the one component that is often overlooked at mealtime, particularly in recipes for salads and snacks. Useful protein boosters are low-fat dairy products; lean meats, poultry and seafood; egg whites; beans; and soy-based foods, such as tofu and isolated soy or whey powders.

BIG-BATCH COOKING SAVES TIME

If you don't always have time to cook, make big batches when you do have time, say, on the weekends, and freeze green-light meals for busy nights. Having healthy meals in your freezer means you can always pull them out rather than grab a takeout menu. With a little planning, you won't have to rely on fast food to get you through your busy schedule. Organizing your pantry, fridge and freezer so that they keep you going when the going gets tough will ensure the weight-loss results you want.

EQUIPMENT

The right equipment will help you gain maximum nutritional benefit as well as save you time. Every G.I. Diet kitchen should have the following:

MICROWAVE OVEN

Heating and cooking foods is really the first step in the digestive process. The longer you cook your food, the more "digestible" it becomes. Ever tried eating a raw potato? It will take you a week to digest it! As a result, cooking raises the G.I. of foods as it does what your tummy would otherwise be doing. Remember, it's important to have your body processing food. Though we don't recommend always eating uncooked foods, we do suggest keeping cooking times to a minimum; or cooking only until, as the Italians say, "al dente" or "with some firmness to the bite."

One of the best ways of doing this is with the microwave oven. Fresh or frozen vegetables can be cooked in minutes and that helps to keep the G.I. low and often preserves nutrients better than other methods, because cooking time is reduced and little water is used. The microwave is a godsend at breakfast as my favourite cereal, oatmeal, can be made in three to four minutes rather than fifteen minutes or more on the stove. A fillet of fish can be cooked in five minutes.

For thawing meats, and warming snacks and leftovers, the microwave is your best green-light kitchen friend.

NONSTICK FRYING PANS

You should have two different sizes plus lids. They require little or no oil, and cleaning up is a cinch. We are big on stir-fries in our household, so these nonstick skillets get a lot of use.

BARBECUES/INDOOR GRILLS

Cooking meat and fish on either a barbecue or indoor grill is a good idea as it allows any extra fat to drain away and the food always seem to taste better too.

E-CLINIC DIARIES

This week e-clinic participants were absorbing the basic information just as you are now.

I wanted to tell you that I hadn't had steel-cut oatmeal since I was a child. (It took me forever to find it, and I had to have my local grocer order it for me!) My Irish grandmother, who lived with us when I was a small child, used to make "porridge" for us every morning before school. My brothers hated it, but I loved it. I never knew that was what she was making, and I couldn't figure out why my quick-cook oatmeal never tasted as good as hers, and so I cut it from my diet over the years. I love the "porridge" and swear I could eat it for every meal, (but won't). I get a truly warm memory when I have it, and think of Grandma stirring that pot of porridge telling us, in her Irish brogue, that "Jesus, Mary and Joseph! If 'twasn't for porridge and the potatoes God gave us, we'd (the Irish) all be dead by now!" If nothing works on this diet, I am grateful for getting that memory back!!! —Carol

Q: Do you really recommend Splenda for a sugar substitute? Do you know anything about stevia or Truvia? I would like to buy something this week which will work and be low–GI. —Gail

A: Splenda is my top choice but you can try stevia (or Truvia, which is the same thing but made by Coca-Cola™), which is a natural sweetener from a South American plant. As I mentioned, I personally I don't like the aftertaste but that's an individual thing.

Q: A naturopath told me that it is silly to pay for omega-3 eggs when all you have to do is use a free-range egg and add ¼ to ½ tsp of flax oil per egg and you will have the very same thing. I am hoping this works, as the only real grumbling I get from my husband is when he sees store-bought eggs in the refrigerator when we have ninety chickens that are free range and fed chicken scratch that has corn, wheat, barley and oats. What's your take on this? —Casey

A: Omega-3 eggs are produced by feeding chickens with flaxseed, which gives their eggs the omega-3 content. So adding flaxseed oil—or ground flax seeds—to the eggs is just fine. I don't blame your husband for grumbling when you have fresh eggs in your backyard!

Q: Can you use a whey protein shake mixed with frozen fruit and skim milk for breakfast? This is what I have been using and I find it quite filling. By the way, as you suggested, I changed to sugar-free, caffeine-free cola and have noticed that my blood sugar level dropped. — Judy

A: One of the principles of the G.I. Diet is to let your tummy do the processing rather than the manufacturer or processor. Blending, in effect, does what your stomach does and thus speeds up digestion, the reverse of what we are trying to achieve. All the ingredients you mention are green-light but I suggest you eat them together unblended except for the protein powder mixed in milk.

Week 2 went well for me. It was my first week to do this diet at home and I lost a small bit of weight even while eating regularly at home. When we were away in week 1, I didn't always fit in all my snacks or all my meals. I am trying to eat slower and enjoy it more and I feel full with less food. I have never lost weight quickly and now, being older, I'm not expecting that I will lose quickly on this weight loss program either. "Slow and steady wins the race" is certainly the way to go for me. I expect that it might take me a year to get all the weight off that I want. That doesn't mean that I'm not impatient! —Trish

Q: I am enjoying this process tremendously. Eating low–G.I. is not difficult and, as important, not eating red-light foods is not difficult. How many pieces of fruit (oranges, grapefruit, apples) can be eaten in one day? I love fruit and am nervous about the fructose. —Gail

A: While I do not place a limit on the quantity of fruit you should consume, I expect you to use common sense and moderation as in all things. Fructose has a relatively low G.I. so that is going to have less impact on your blood sugar levels than regular sugar. However, fructose still contains the same number of calories as sugar, so eating an excessive amount of fruit will not help to reduce those pounds.

By now you should be getting more comfortable with cooking and eating the green-light way. Next week we will be focusing on the single most important factor in successful weight loss: portion control.

For Week 2, please see optional meal plan B on pages 177–180 in Part 4.

Week 2 Weight: _____

Week 2 Waist: _____

WEEK 2 DIARY

_____

_____

_____

_____

_____

_____

_____

_____

_____

_____

_____

Week 3
Portion Distortion

Reducing weight and controlling blood sugar levels is a combination of what you eat and how much. By now, most people will be feeling comfortable with the basic principles of eating the green-light way. Making the right food choices is not as difficult as you thought! However, it's still all too easy to trip up over the question of how much you should eat and jeopardize your weight-loss results.

One of the principal reasons that we have an obesity crisis is the size of servings and portions. A serving size is what is recommended whereas a portion size is what you choose to eat. We have undergone a radical change in our perception of portion sizes over the past twenty years or so, principally because of the super-sizing of fast-food and family restaurant meals during this time. These have now become our serving-size norms in what is described as "portion distortion." Let me give you some examples with a list prepared by the U.S. National Heart, Lung and Blood Institute:

	20 YEARS AGO		TODAY	
	Size	Calories	Size	Calories
SNACKS				
Bagel	3 inches	140	6 inches	350
French fries	2.4 ounces	210	7 ounces	610
Muffin	1.5 ounces	210	5 ounces	500
Cookie	1 ½ inches	55	4 inches	275
MEALS				
Spaghetti and meatballs		500		1025
Turkey sandwich		320		820
Chicken Caesar salad		390		700
Chicken stir-fry		435		865

As you can see, the size and corresponding calories have doubled or even trebled over this relatively short time period. These new sizes have become today's serving norms and that translates into how you see portions on your plate. No wonder there's "portion distortion" and ballooning waistlines. Does this mean that we were all starving in the disco era—or are we simply eating more now because it's there?

Last September I was diagnosed with type 2 diabetes and was given 3 months to loose a significant amount of weight. After three months, I was to have a blood test (HBA1C) to determine if medication was required to keep me well.

After doing some research on the internet, I found your website and ordered your book. I found it easy to read and liked that it explained how the low G.I. program actually worked. I am a person who needs to understand how something works before I am able to move forward with the program.

I am pleased to say that in the first 3 months I lost 35 lbs and do not require any medication. The weight has continued to fall off me with very little effort. I don't feel like I have been on a diet, and though I miss some foods, such as cheese (in the quantaties I used to eat it), I have not felt short changed or deprived.

I have now lost just over 55 lbs and am finding myself much more active and feeling very well. The gym is no longer a chore and everyday activities take half the time as they used to. Even the dog has lost 10 lbs! I still have 40 lbs to loose and am just about to have repeat blood tests done again, but I'm not expecting any nasty surprises.

I now have the full collection of your books and, with your advice and recipes, I have enjoyed my new lifestyle program.

Thank you once again.

Nicky

A study done of college students on their consumption of their favourite food, macaroni and cheese, shows that the more that was put in front of them, the more they ate (if the food was there, they ate it). Yet they reported that they felt no fuller on the larger portions than they felt with the smaller ones! Moral: if it's not on your plate, you won't miss it.

To further reinforce the message, when researchers were trying to discover why the French are far less obese than Americans, they compared similar eateries in Paris and Philadelphia. They found the average serving size was 25 percent greater in Philadelphia. In supermarkets a similar pattern emerged with fourteen of seventeen items larger in the U.S. stores (e.g., candy bars, 41 percent larger; soft drinks, 52 percent larger; hot dogs, 63 percent larger; and yoghurt, 82 percent larger.

Though most of us have been aware of the super-sizing of foods in recent years, what we don't realize is that this portion distortion has slipped into home-prepared meals too. To make it easier to reduce our green-light portions, especially as no one likes to weigh and measure foods, here are some ways of eyeballing your portion sizes using familiar objects:

½ cup breakfast cereal . . . . ½ baseball

½ tsp margarine . . . . top half of thumb

4 oz meat . . . . palm of your hand

4 oz fish . . . . small hot dog bun

¾ cup pasta (cooked) . . . . size of your fist

⅔ cup rice (cooked) . . . . one tennis ball

Although we don't recommend particular serving sizes for most green-light foods, we do stress moderation and common sense. For example, typical servings should be

Fruit (e.g., an apple) equals a tennis ball.
Vegetable (e.g., broccoli) equals a lightbulb.
Dairy product (e.g., cottage cheese) equals half a hardball.

Here are some helpful tips for watching those serving sizes:

- Don't eat in front of the TV as you will be unaware of how much food you've eaten.
- Eat slowly as it takes 20 to 30 minutes for the message to get from your tummy to your brain. Put down your fork/spoon between mouthfuls.
- Divide your plate into three:

  - One-quarter for meat/fish/chicken/tofu.
  - One-quarter for rice/potatoes/pasta.
  - One-half for vegetables (a minimum of two).

- Don't snack from a bag (e.g., count out a serving of nuts and put them into a bowl).
- Ask for small servings when eating out, or split an entree with your companion.

Soon you will look back aghast at the amount you used to eat. I look around restaurants today when dining out and never cease to be amazed at what people can put away in a sitting!

E-CLINIC DIARIES

Week 3 found many of the e-clinic participants getting into the swing of reducing their serving sizes with some interesting side effects:

> *For the most part my blood sugars are greatly improved and I cut my night dose of Lantus by 3 units, from 25 to 22. . . . My glucose machine showed me a day into this eating [plan] that my average 30-day reading was 9.9 and that is down to 8.7. Day 14 was 8.9 and is now down to 7.0. Most of my readings have been below 5.5 [since then].* —Sharon

> *Q: What is the difference between the glycemic index and the glycemic load I have heard about? How does the glycemic load impact on weight loss and sugar control?* —Joanne

> A: Glycemic load is a formula that takes into account the number of carbohydrates in a given food as well as its glycemic index rating. This is one of the factors taken into account when foods are rated on the traffic-light-colour scale. The whole concept behind the traffic-light system was to simplify the food selection process by doing all the calculations as to glycemic index/load, fat levels and calories for you.

> *I am doing ok with all your recommendations. Have cut out all pastries and watching sweets very closely. My blood sugar is good. That is a plus. However, I'm having a difficult time cutting out the wine and drinks at cocktail hour (after all, I am down south at the moment!). I have started enjoying virgin Caesars . . . I try to keep it to two glasses of wine per night. Will try and work on one glass per night for the coming week. Will have to start measuring and*

weighing my food at dinner time because I know that my portions are a little big for what I should be eating. —Helene

"She who must be obeyed" was rummaging through my overfull bag of garbage in my car when she discovered my empty pumpkin seed bag. When I bought them I was overjoyed to read that the seeds contained 25 grams of fibre. When my wife discovered the empty bag, she asked me, "Did you eat the whole bag at one sitting?" Yes. "Well, you just ate 500 calories." Hmm. Why are "they" always right? —John

Q: For the most part I can visualize how much I should be eating, but some things still are questionable. For example, should I be eating a whole can of tuna or salmon (213 g) at one sitting? It seems like a lot. —Barb

A: A serving of meat, fish or chicken should be no more than 120 grams or 4 ounces. You are serving yourself close to twice that amount. Get into the habit of checking your portion servings against the twelve specific green-light serving size recommendations listed on page 25. These green-light food listings have been selected deliberately because they all have the potential to add a lot of extra unnecessary calories if the serving sizes are exceeded. In most other cases you can eat as much green-light food as you like, providing you use moderation and common sense.

It was interesting reading about increasing portion sizes. I find I'm going the other way! Yesterday I thawed out the Chicken Jambalaya for lunch and couldn't eat it all—it was even less than a full portion. But I was hungry for my snack at three so felt satisfied. I went with a group for Chinese dinner last Saturday and slipped somewhat, but since it was my only error all week I was happy with my results. My fasting blood sugar is up and down every day, but the average is around 6, so that's good. I saw my doctor yesterday and he noticed the weight loss. I showed him your book (amazingly enough he had not heard about it) and told him I couldn't wait to get my next A1C done! —Ade

Q: What is your opinion of fasting or liquid fasting one day a week? I have read that this is beneficial. —Howard

A: I have little time for fasting, liquid fasting or any crash diets as they are only temporary expedients that camouflage the fact that that you fundamentally have to change your eating habits permanently if you are to lose weight and keep it off. Fasting may well lead to short-term weight loss but it is rarely sustainable and interferes with adopting the healthy eating behaviours that are essential to long-term success. Inevitably you will find yourself starving after the fast and you will overeat for a while as your body regains its equilibrium. Fasting is also unhealthy and even dangerous for anyone with diabetes. Remember the G.I. Diet is not a short-term diet, but rather a new way of eating that will continue for the rest of your life.

You are doing extremely well on this program and will continue to do so providing you don't get deflected by the false promises of miracle weight loss that surround us.

Having now dealt with both what you should be eating and how much, next week we will be examining the other principal cause of weight gain, your own eating behaviours. This is a subject that gets scant attention in many books on weight control yet it is absolutely critical to your eventual success.

For Week 3, please see optional meal plan B on pages 177–180 in Part 4.

Week 3 Weight: _____

Week 3 Waist: _____

WEEK 3 DIARY

_____

_____

_____

_____

_____

Week 4
Behaviour Change

This week we will discuss arguably the most important long-term component in this clinic: behaviour change. Read the following carefully, and then reread it because it will have a long-term impact on your success. By the time you are diagnosed as diabetic or pre-diabetic, your lifestyle patterns and personal habits are well established. Over the years you have made choices that, for better or worse, have deeply entrenched your food habits. And change, once so welcome in youth, is much more difficult to embrace. However, changing behaviours with regard to food is fundamental to your success with this program.

This week we will examine some behaviours that must be addressed. Some of you may well have already changed some of these behaviours, but there will be others, which out of ignorance or choice, have become part of your life. I can provide you with the tools to change what you eat but changing your food behaviours is something that only you can do. As the old saying goes, "You can lead a horse to water, but you cannot make it drink"!

Here are ten important behaviours that must be addressed if you are to be successful in reaching your weight-loss goals.

1. SKIPPING BREAKFAST

This is a very common bad habit: it is estimated that one-quarter of North Americans skip breakfast, and the numbers are even worse for teenagers.

Breakfast is the most important meal of the day. By the time people rise in the morning, most haven't eaten for ten to twelve hours, and their blood sugar levels are low. As a result, skipping breakfast will most certainly cause you to snack throughout the day in an effort to boost your blood sugar or energy level. At the end of the day, chances are you'll be starving and unnecessarily stuffing yourself at dinner. Neither of these activities will help stabilize blood sugar levels or shrink your waistline.

2. NOT TAKING TIME TO EAT PROPERLY

Saying "I don't have time to eat properly" creates a spawning ground for bad habits. People who don't take the time to eat properly tend to nibble their way through the day usually on high-fat, high-sugar snacks, pick up some high-fat takeout food on the way home for dinner, and finally collapse in front of the TV for the evening with beer and a bowl of chips.

It's easy to slip into this harmful cycle of fattening convenience food and short-term energy fixes, but you'll pay for the convenience with erratic blood sugar levels, a growing girth, flagging energy and poor health. And really, the amount of time required to prepare your own healthy meals and snacks is quite modest. Fifteen minutes in the morning is all it takes to eat a healthy breakfast—often the length of time it takes to line up for a coffee. If you can't manage to wake up fifteen minutes earlier to squeeze in a nutritious breakfast before rushing off to work, then bring along a box of green-light cereal, a carton of skim milk and a piece of fruit. Another piece of fruit and a carton of skim milk take no time to prepare and makes a filling, nutritious snack. And there are always places you can get a green-light sandwich so you don't have to resort to pizza. Eating healthily through the day will ensure that you have the energy when you arrive home to prepare a quick green-light dinner in the time it would have taken to drive to the takeout place and wait for your order.

3. GRAZING

The world's best grazers are teenagers. They simply cannot avoid opening the fridge every time they pass it. Their rapid growth and (hopefully) high activity levels require a constant high-calorie intake. Unfortunately, grazing is a habit that many people continue into their adult lives with disastrous results for their waistlines and health. A few nuts here, a couple of cookies there, a tablespoon or two of peanut butter, and a few glasses of juice all look pretty harmless in themselves, but taken together they can easily total several hundred extra calories a day! And those can add up to over 20 pounds of additional weight in a year.

On the G.I. Diet, you should be eating three meals plus three to four snacks a day, which means you are eating approximately every two to three hours or so during your waking hours. This will reduce your temptation to graze. One reader wrote that she couldn't believe how she could be losing weight when she always seemed to be eating. She called it "green-light grazing"!

4. UNCONSCIOUS EATING

How often have we all begun to nibble on a bowl of chips or nuts or a box of cookies while watching TV, reading a book or talking on the phone and then suddenly realized that we'd eaten the whole lot. Too often, I would guess.

Eating should never be the peripheral activity—it should always be the focus. Eat your meals at the table and set aside distractions such as the TV, computer, video game or telephone while you have your snacks. This will help you to always eat consciously and be aware of exactly how much you are eating.

5. EATING TOO QUICKLY

The famous Dr. Johnson of the eighteenth century is said to have asserted that food should always be chewed thirty-two times before swallowing. Though this seems rather excessive, there is an important truth here. Many of us tend to eat far too quickly. It takes 20–30 minutes for the stomach to let the brain know it is full. If you eat too quickly, you'll continue to eat past the point at which you've had enough. The solution, then, is to eat slowly to allow the brain to catch up with your stomach.

That's probably another reason that Mediterranean countries have lower rates of obesity: they take far longer to eat their meals. A recent report showed the French taking twice as long over their meals as Canadians. In France, mealtimes are for family and friends, for enjoying the pleasure of food—not simply a means to tackle hunger. To ensure you are not eating more than your appetite requires, slow down and really enjoy what you are eating. Put your fork down between mouthfuls. Savour the flavours and textures.

6. NOT DRINKING ENOUGH

Did you know that by the time you feel thirsty you are already dehydrated? Your body's need for water is second only to its need for oxygen. Up to 70 percent of the body is water, and we should be drinking about eight glasses of fluid a day to replenish our supply. Fluids include water, milk, coffee/tea and soft drinks. Yet many of us don't take the time to drink enough, and we think we are tired and hungry, which makes us reach for food when we really should be reaching for a glass of water. Our body isn't hungry, it's thirsty. So make sure you are drinking your eight glasses. Being properly hydrated will go a long way toward helping you control your appetite and lose weight.

7. REWARDING FOR EXERCISE

Another common habit is rewarding yourself with food for doing some exercise. Rather than allowing the reward to be the exercise itself, many feel that the extra effort deserves some form of reward or treat, which more often than not takes the form of food or drink.

This raises a couple of issues. First, one of the great myths about weight loss is that it can be achieved through exercise alone. Though exercise is essential for long-term health and weight maintenance, it is actually a poor tool for losing weight. To give you an idea of how much exercise you would have to do to lose just one pound of fat, you would have to walk briskly for 42 miles if you weighed 160 pounds or 53 miles if you weighed 130 pounds. That is a huge amount of effort and way beyond the capability or time availability of most people. Walking around the block or washing the car consumes only a handful of calories. So if you are using exercise as permission to cut a little slack in your diet, remember that cookie reward will add more calories than you expended on your activity.

By all means, exercise to improve your health, but don't think it will significantly contribute to your weight loss. I frequently tell people that losing weight is 90 percent diet and 10 percent exercise, particularly in the early stages.

8. CLEANING THE PLATE

Many of us were taught from the time we were small to finish what's on our plates before leaving the table. This becomes a deeply embedded habit that does not, unfortunately, help us in later life to lose or maintain weight. Not only do we finish our own, but we tend to also finish the leftovers on our children's plates or that last lonely slice in the pie dish after dinner. But this habit causes us to eat more than we need to satisfy our hunger and is therefore dreadful for weight control. Get into the habit of letting your stomach and brain decide when you are full, not the quantity of food on your plate. Leftovers can always be stored in the fridge, rather than around your waist or hips.

9. SHOPPING ON AN EMPTY STOMACH

Human nature can often be perverse, encouraging us to do the right thing but at the wrong time. When you are full and satisfied, food shopping is rarely top of mind. But when you are hungry, grocery shopping suddenly seems like a very good idea indeed. Unfortunately, it isn't: you'll end up with a shopping cart that has been filled primarily by your stomach rather than your head. Those red-light foods will seem far more tempting than usual, and you will probably make some poor choices as a result.

So always shop after a meal, or at least take a green-light snack such as a muffin or a nutrition bar with you. You'll make far wiser choices this way.

10. EATING HIGH-SUGAR, HIGH-FAT TREATS

As we are all aware, food is a big part of holidays and celebrations—just think of Thanksgiving, a wedding, a bar mitzvah or Christmas and you'll probably picture the special foods that go along with them. Where would the candy industry be without birthdays, Valentine's Day, Halloween or Easter? Food is inexorably linked with positive experiences, and that is one of reasons we often think of certain foods as "treats." Whether it's Granny doling out candies to a child who has been good, or a neighbour presenting you with a freshly baked pie as reward for raking up her leaves, we are accustomed to using food treats to reward the people in our lives as well as ourselves. Unfortunately, these so-called treats tend to be high in calories, sugar and fat and are certainly not your friends. They are a major contributor to the obesity crisis and to weight-related diseases such as diabetes and heart disease. We should start to view these foods as penalties rather than rewards.

Instead, choose treats that are lower in calories and fat. If candy is your thing, there is a plethora of low- and no-sugar brands available. Fresh fruit, low-fat, no-sugar-added yogurt and ice cream are even better treats. And there are many delicious green-light dessert and snack recipes in all my G.I. Diet books. Treats are a wonderful part of our lives—just make sure they are the right sort of treats.

Five months ago I was diagnosed as insulin resistant or pre-diabetic. I was introduced to the low-glycemic diet [G.I. Diet] by a friend and read all the [G.I.] books. I now have lost 40 pounds and am at a normal BMI. My blood sugars are in a normal range. I will not go back to any other way of eating. I look around now at what other people eat and see how our society has really let things get out of hand in terms of unhealthy eating. Hopefully this way of eating will reach many more people before they are faced with diabetes and other health-related issues.

Thank you,
Bett Anne

Keep in mind that while it will take some effort and can be challenging at times to change old bad habits, it's well worth your while to persevere with beneficial new behaviours. Before you know it, they'll be second nature, new habits as firmly entrenched as old ones used to be. But these ones will help slim down to a brand-new you.

E- CLINIC DIARIES

As the clinic participants continued on their weight-loss journey, some were disappointed by the results. On a positive note, there were moments of self-recognition about how habits have changed as they have adapted to the G.I. Diet:

Changing entrenched behaviours is a biggy for me. I am a nibbler and have got to stop that impulse. The food is in my mouth and I'm chewing before I realize. I am going to try to be more conscious this week. We are heading to a resort for a few days, so restaurant eating lies ahead. I am determined to try to make good choices. Going to make sure I bring some healthy snacks with me so I'm not too hungry at meals. —Shannon

It's been a bit of a trying week just based on family issues. However, the G.I. Diet is not putting on any extra-added stress. It is making me think about food choices more—and think of the money I'm saving by not eating out as often!! It certainly has made me realize how much we tend to overeat/nibble without needing to. —Donna

I haven't lost as much as I might have this week because of two dinners out related to work, goodies that are made by my students . . . and my throwing a birthday party for my twins, which involved ice cream, chocolate cake, pizza, lasagne, garlic bread—all their favourites. Mind you, there was also salad and raw veggies and hummus, so I did have an out. Life intrudes constantly and strains the best of intentions. If I have to indulge (and sometimes I have to avoid hurt feelings) I try to have just a tiny bit. Still, I feel that I'm sabotaging my efforts when I do this and risk going whole hog. After all, I reason, this day is ruined, so I may as well enjoy myself. This is a way of thinking that has dogged me all my life, and I know that I have to shake it once and for all. —Kate

I find that often I get caught driving in the car at noontime not close to home and start to get hungry. In former times I would rush into the closest fast-food drive-in and grab a burger or anything to stop the hunger. Now I am starting to remember to pack some almonds, a Balance Bar or a berry muffin, and water, and am planning better for the day, just in case, to hold me over. One wouldn't leave home with your baby or doggie without a snack and water, so why not think about yourself in the same way! Also I keep a very small copy of the green-light foods list with me just as a little reminder of what I can eat if I do have to stop to eat. —Chandra*

I was a wee bit disappointed when I weighed and measured myself this morning and sneaky thoughts like, well, maybe I'll wait till tomorrow to send my stats in popped into my head, but then I checked my blood sugar and was thrilled with that number. I was thinking that at this rate it will take forever to get the weight off. Then the light bulb went on. What difference does it make—if this is how I'm going to eat for the rest of my life, the weight will come off gradually. Like Trish, another clinic member, says, "slow and steady wins the race." I must keep that foremost in my mind. —Karen*

Changing bad habits can be a challenge no matter how old you are! Check off the ones that you have already addressed and focus on those you know need attending to. Don't try to change them all at once or you will get frustrated and give up. Next week we will look at how to maintain those new eating habits and keep your motivation high.

For Week 4, please see optional meal plan B on pages 177–180 in Part 4.

Week 4 Weight: _____

Week 4 Waist: _____

WEEK 4 DIARY

_____

_____

_____

_____

_____

_____

_____

_____

_____

_____

_____

_____

_____

_____

_____

_____

_____

_____

_____

Week 5
Keeping Motivated

At this point, some people may have taken to the G.I. Diet like the proverbial duck to water; however, others have struggled to make the transition from their red-light habits to the green-light way of eating. Regardless of what camp you are in, this is a good time to reflect upon what can be done to keep your motivation high.

It's likely that your struggle with diabetes and its effect on your health is the first and most important motivator for going on the G.I. Diet. For those of you who take your blood sugar readings regularly, it's possible that these may have shown improvement by now. For those of you on medication, you may be talking with your doctor about reducing your medication if those blood sugar readings continue to improve. To become medication free can become a realistic objective for many. It can mean lower prescription costs and fewer side effects. What could be more motivating!

However, on a day-to-day basis, especially during those times when you feel you are not making enough progress or your stress levels become overwhelming, motivation can take a battering. Many of you have work and home and unrelated health pressures that have complicated matters. You wouldn't be human if you didn't feel your resolve starting to waver occasionally. When it does, there are a number of things you can do to encourage yourself to keep going.

1. REMEMBER YOUR INITIAL REASONS.
Reread your reasons for wanting to lose weight in Week 1 (see page 57). Remember why it was so important to you to slim down when you started this journey, and why you need to persevere.

2. USE PHYSICAL REMINDERS OF YOUR GOAL.
Keep a picture of an outfit you're going to buy when you reach your goal, or a photograph of a thinner you where you will see it every day. One reader, who is blind, kept a picture in her mind's eye. She told me "I am using my beautiful red leather coat as the motivator for me. Last winter when I went to put it on, it was about two inches too small. I was not able to close the zipper. Now when I put the coat on, I

am able to zip up the coat. Tight yes, but I know that I have made progress. What an incredible feeling. What motivation for me . . . I am determined to wear the coat this winter."

3. KEEP IN MIND HOW FAR YOU'VE COME.

Compare yourself now to where you were before you started the diet. How much weight have you lost? How much better do your clothes fit you? How has your energy level and health improved? What can you do now that you couldn't do before? Going back to your old eating habits won't seem so tempting when you think how it will undermine all the good things that weight loss has brought you so far.

> *I have Type II diabetes. Your book has changed my life and my understanding about eating. I started following your suggested food plan and I have lost 27 pounds and am still losing. In the past everything I ate gave me that diabetic flush and that dazed feeling. It never failed, around two o'clock in the afternoon I always felt tired and miserable. Someone told me that was all part of being a diabetic. I got to the point in my life I was always going off my diet, falling off the wagon and getting that cruddy feeling that affects thousands that are in the same boat as me.*
>
> *Thank you. Your book is very well written and easy to understand.*
> *Richard*
> *P.S. This is the best I've felt in 10 years!*

4. THE SHOPPING BAG MOTIVATOR

Often people don't realize how much weight actually weighs. Sounds crazy, but when people tell me they've lost only 20 pounds, I ask them to fill a couple of shopping bags with 20 pounds of books and carry them up and down the stairs a few times. Everyone is always glad to put the bags down and report they had no idea how heavy 20 pounds really is.

So the next time you're feeling uninspired, fill a shopping bag or two with the amount of books or cans of food that equals how much weight you've lost since you started the program and carry them up and down a flight of stairs three times. You'll be amazed at what you've lost, and you'll be relieved to put the bag down. You couldn't have put that weight down weeks ago when it was still around your waist, hips and thighs.

One lady used potatoes for weight and when the bag reached 40 pounds she couldn't even lift it, let alone walk around with it. She had absolutely no idea this is what she had been carrying around for years. "No wonder," she wrote, "I lacked energy and my back and knees were always sore!"

In a previous e-clinic, several members found this incentive very motivating and suggested filling empty bottles with water equivalent to the weight they lost each week. One member went further and filled bottles with water equivalent to the weight she intended to lose, placing them on one side of her scale. She placed empty bottles on the other side and transferred water over each week equivalent to the weekly amount of weight she had lost. Both of these ideas struck me as a simple and flexible idea way to remind yourself visually of your progress.

5. GET SUPPORT.

Buddy up with friends, a spouse or family members who are trying to lose weight. They will give you a sense of camaraderie and encouragement as you strive for your goal, and you can turn to them for support when you need it.

6. THE $10 CURE.

This is a motivator that people often stumble upon by accident. The siren song of a red-light lunch draws them into a fast-food chain, where they order a burger with the works, a large french fries and a shake. Mid-afternoon, they feel lousy and can barely keep their eyes open. They've found out the hard way where straying from the green-light gets you.

I call this the $10 cure because it's the food version of what immigrants (like me!) used to call the $1,000 cure. Whenever a new arrival, after a long cold winter in Canada, used to pine for the "old country," the cure was to get on a plane and go home for a week. All the reasons that originally persuaded the person to emigrate would come crashing back, and the thought of flying back to Canada would begin to look pretty good again.

With food, the cure costs less—says $10 (maybe $15 with inflation!). But this is a motivator of last resort only; I certainly don't want to encourage people to abuse their bodies and feel awful! However, if you've been unceasingly pining for red-light foods, go out for lunch with some friends and order that burger, fries and a shake. Your mouth may enjoy it, but I guarantee that a couple of hours later you'll be regretting the deviation.

E-CLINIC DIARIES

Motivation comes in many forms, whether it's one of the coping strategies I've outlined above, a change in your blood sugar readings or simply the knowledge that while it didn't happen this week, if you keep at it, the weight loss will come. Take a moment to think about what motivates you while you are on this journey. Here are some thoughts from our e-clinic participants on the subject:

I am trying to listen more to my body and feel the fullness during a meal. I'm eating things with more crunch that require lots of chewing and take longer to eat. A nice hot cup of tea finishes off the meal and makes me feel full. Then a while later if I feel hungry again I tell myself that I couldn't be hungry, since I ate only an hour ago. I give it time to let the feeling go away. I keep busy with other things. I get anxious when I'm hungry, so I'm trying to let that feeling go. Also, I have a couple of my own behaviour changes that I'd like to share with you.

1. I make sure I don't get too hungry between eating times as this tends to trigger eating too much at one sitting and for me that leads to weight gain even if I eat the green-light foods . . . I really need to keep my portions small for me to lose weight. I always try to take green-light snacks with me, but sometimes it's hard to have them when I get too busy. I'm working on it!

2. And I continually keep reading about the proper way to eat in order to keep my motivation at a high level. If I let a few days go by without reading some green-light recipes or parts of the [G.I. Diet] books, it gets too easy to start thinking the old ways. If I read the books and study the lists, I do much better and feel more confident. —Trish

I have done rather well this week. Each week, I try to work on making a small change to my routine. (Don't they say that new behaviours practised regularly for at least six to eight weeks start becoming ingrained as habits?)

My first week, I tried to get up every time a commercial came on TV in the evening and did SOMETHING. It's amazing how many commercials there are in one 30-minute program! So, in other words, I moved my body when I would ordinarily just sit there. I often did 3 minutes' worth of laundry or some dusting or vacuuming but stayed out of the kitchen.

The second week, I stopped all eating after 8:00 pm.

The third week, when I was on yard duty, I walked the perimeter of the playground—through deep snow, which is quite a workout.

The fourth and fifth weeks, I was on holidays and just held on to the new habits I had already started.

I find that a daily read of your information helps me to keep focused. I also find that going to bed earlier (i.e., by 10:00) gets me out of harm's way. I am up by 6:00, do not feel like eating yet and thus spend the extra hour till 7:00 being active around the house. That way, the hour is spent far more productively at the beginning of the day rather than at the end. In fact, I am going to count this as my new habit in the coming week! —Kate

I grew up a skinny runner, and stayed active until my early 30s when my kids were in school. I went back to an office job and the pounds crept on. I stayed thin with Weight Watchers, but the weighing and measuring and strictness of the diet back in the late 70s was brutal, so I rebelled and went from 120 pounds to a high of 230 pounds over a 15 to 20–year term. That's why this is so good: no food diaries, no serving-size restrictions, and no hunger; sometimes I have to remind myself to eat, can you imagine that?! My husband is also amazed; he watches his diet due to sodium and saturated fats so we are in this together! I bought a book to give to my daughter who is starting to struggle with weight gain, and I have several friends who are interested. My blood sugar levels have been well under 6 all week, so my average for the week is about 5.5—love it! I will get an A1C in a week or two; my doctor doesn't know about this yet and will be so happy! So again I shout from the rooftop, THANK YOU, RICK! —Ade

YAHOO! I am so excited about this way of eating. I have cut my Metformin in half and my blood sugar is still wonderful . . . My dream is to be off diabetic medication completely by the time we finish the e-clinic. I think that each week also brings along lessons with it. Twice now I have gone to a Spanish class expecting to be home on time to have a snack and lunch. Because I started late, the instructor invited me for some private tutoring, and being the people pleaser that I am I could not say no. In fact, I really wanted the extra help—but I had no snack and no lunch because I expected to be home. Of course, it leaves me famished and in dangerous territory. On the way home today I thought, "What's the matter with you—just bring a couple of muffins along and if this situation comes up again you can just have that and if not, you can always bring them home to have later." Now I know what I will do for the next class. I just feel really grateful for being a participant in this clinic and pray that my frame of mind will stay where it is now. I have many times experienced success for 20 to 25 pounds and then I just seem to lose it. I think this might be different because I do not feel hungry or deprived of things I really like and crave. —Corinne

Motivators? Hmm . . . I know that when my stomach growls out of hunger, especially late in the evening, I tell myself that is the feeling of weight being lost at that moment. I like to imagine some little Pac-Man–like cells nibbling away on my fat! Because evenings are my worst time to succumb to temptations, I have taped some weight-loss TV shows (X-weighted, Biggest Loser) and I go up to my bedroom where we have a TV, crawl into bed and watch other people lose weight! Nothing motivates me like seeing someone else be successful, because I tend to be "just a bit" competitive (that last is written with tongue firmly in cheek).

Using the power of my mind and imagination is one way I keep myself motivated. I like to conjure up images of myself being fit and healthy, slim and trim. I picture myself in white tennis shorts and a sleeveless top playing singles with my husband. I see myself running a 5K with my kids or in a bathing suit on the beach. Mental pictures and visual pictures too (the photo of me on my fridge when I was slim and trim) help me to keep focused.

Chewing sugar-free gum sometimes helps, because my mouth is moving. Sometimes brushing and flossing my teeth right after I eat puts a note of finality to the meal and prevents me from nibbling while I clean up the kitchen. I know this is not for everyone, but going to the gym (I just joined) makes me feel virtuous and totally motivated the minute I walk in the door. Any little bit of exercise is fantastic for the feeling of doing something good for yourself. —Kate

Carrying the bag of weight equal to what I have lost is the best pat on the back I have found. Makes me feel good about myself and motivated to keep on trying. —Pat

Staying motivated is crucial to successful weight loss. It keeps you focused and on the green-light path and it will get you through the pitfalls you'll encounter. Next week we'll get some tips from my wife, Dr. Ruth Gallop, an expert in behaviour, on how many of us use food as a way to comfort ourselves during stressful times.

For Week 5, please see optional meal plan B on pages 177-180 in Part 4.

Week 5 Weight: _____

Week 5 Waist: _____

WEEK 5 DIARY

_____

_____

_____

_____

_____

_____

_____

_____

_____

_____

_____

_____

Week 6
Food for Comfort

This week we will address the issue of emotional eating, frequently described as using "food for comfort." I have asked my wife, Dr. Ruth Gallop, Professor Emeritus at the University of Toronto, to write this section, as one of her specialties is childhood trauma and how that plays out in adult life. This has given her considerable insight into the whole question of the role of food in helping people deal with their emotional issues. We realize that this is a very large topic but hope to provide you with some guidance. Here are some of her thoughts:

When we have reasonably balanced lives, food plays an important but not dominant role in our day-to-day lives. When our lives are out of balance and we don't feel good about certain aspects of our lives, then food can take over. When we don't feel good about ourselves and experience low self-esteem, food can be a powerful and damaging force. This is particularly true for women. Women live in a society fixated on how we should look. Putting aside all the healthy reasons for being at a "normal" weight, our society just doesn't approve of big people. And, more importantly, big people often don't approve of themselves.

Frequently, eating to feel better is preceded by negative feelings. For some people these feelings may include sadness, loneliness or even boredom. For others the feelings can be more in the range of anger, irritability or high stress. These feelings can lead to a vicious eating cycle. It goes something like this:

I feel: depressed; angry; bored; sad; bad about myself (low self-esteem) ⤳ so I eat to feel better ⤳ I experience a brief blood sugar high and feel better ⤳ I experience a blood sugar crash and feel terrible ⤳ I feel bad about myself for eating, for failing ⤳ so I eat to feel better . . . and around I go.

In many situations the original reasons for feeling bad about oneself or getting angry, overwhelmed or disappointed may have origins in our childhood; overeating, negative body image and low self-esteem are the current consequence. Usually we do not make any conscious link between past events and current behaviour. For example, as a child, parental approval/love may have been connected with food via treats or eating all that was put in front of us. Or we may have been punished (by withdrawal of love) if we didn't eat our vegetables! Eating becomes connected to trying to recapture that good feeling of being loved. Although we are unaware of these motives or psychological reasons for the behaviour, we have done it for so long it becomes part of our food and eating habits.

Rick's mother cannot bear to see food that is on the table unfinished regardless of whether or not a person is still hungry. At ninety-nine years of age she still says, "I do like to see a clean plate" when all the food on the table has disappeared. I have learned to deal with this learned behaviour—a behaviour that earned Rick love and approval from his mother—by never putting excess food on the table at mealtimes or making up the dinner plates before I serve them. I don't put out bowls of food for individual selection; otherwise, Rick will unconsciously graze on a lot of extra food!

If you are ready to change your eating habits, the first thing to do is to become aware of them. For example, every time you walk in the front door, is the first stop the fridge or cookie cupboard? When you have had a bad day, do you deal with it by eating something sweet or creamy? When you feel bored and have nothing structured to do, do you eat? Are you unable to watch TV without food in your hand so that you end up eating more than you realize unconsciously? I have one piece of dark chocolate most evenings if I am watching TV. The other night I realized I was in the middle of eating a second piece with no memory of reaching down and picking it up!

We all eat for comfort. When we are sick, many of us have favourite foods— often foods from our childhood that we associate with being looked after. There are foods we eat rarely and foods we could eat every day—often foods that make us feel good, satiated or even happy.

I bought your book on an impulse a few months ago and after spending two weeks studying and reading it, my husband and I decided the plan looked doable. I have Type II diabetes, hypertension and I'm more than 100 pounds overweight. My husband had recently tested for high cholesterol and needed to lose 25 pounds or so. We emptied our fridge and pantry over a period of time and, armed with your excellent shopping guide, bought most of what we thought we'd need for the first week of the diet.

My husband has lost 20 pounds and a couple of inches . . . I have lost 14 pounds and a few inches around my waist BUT the most remarkable thing is *the normalization of my sugars. My sugars ranged from 14 to 23 with big swings from low to high and vice versa. From the second day, my sugars started dropping and staying more even throughout the day. As a result, I started dropping the amount of insulin I took, very slowly, and checking my sugar levels very carefully. My doctor says if things continue this way, I may be able to go off insulin completely. During my checkup last week we discovered that my blood pressure was normal for the first time in years. This is the first time that I have not felt hungry while trying to lose weight. Thank you for making it relatively easy for a lot of desperate people to quietly try something and succeed.* —Margie*

Take a day or two to jot down your patterns and work out when automatic behaviours take over and when it is most difficult for you to avoid eating in excess. It is important to recognize high-risk situations. Bad habits include

- Grazing—a teenage habit that many have not grown out of,
- Eating when stressed, angry, irritable, tired or frustrated,
- Eating when sad, bored or lonely,
- Eating too quickly—remember, it takes twenty to thirty minutes for the stomach to tell the brain it is full,
- Eating unconsciously—especially in front of the TV or at the movies,
- Eating portions that are far too large. Thanks to fast food and restaurants, many portion sizes have doubled and we have brought this portion distortion into our homes,
- Keeping red-light snacks in your desk drawer to eat when you are stressed at work,
- Always eating during any social activity, whether it's sports events, a social visit or even just walking with a friend.

If food comforts you when you are stressed, or when you set unrealistic expectations for yourself, such as getting the household and family errands done, cooking all the meals, or looking after aged parents, then recognize these patterns so you can consider alternative ways to cope, such as sharing tasks with others.

Once you are aware of how comfort eating plays a role in your life, you can begin to change your eating behaviour. You have already taken the first step by making sure that all the food in your house and workplace, as well as all food going into your mouth, is green-light. Reward yourself for this accomplishment. Do something nice for yourself—a little treat like a new lipstick, makeup or perfume—just make sure it isn't red-light food!

Start by trying to modify your behaviours one at a time. If you usually walk in the front door and eat a snack, make sure it is one of your snack times and you have a green-light snack at the ready.

It is particularly important to have snacks with a good, sweet mouth feel when sugar cravings take over. Fruit muffins (use raspberries, blueberries, strawberries or peaches) make an excellent sweet snack as do fresh berries sweetened with Splenda and perhaps served with a dollop of Splenda-sweetened non-fat sour cream. Even sugar-free candies are better than a red-light chocolate bar. Sugar cravings will lessen as long as you stick with green-light foods, and eat three meals and three snacks a day.

Make a list of pleasurable activities you could be doing instead of eating. For example, if you sit in front of the TV and eat, what else could you be doing? Many people like to do something while watching TV; I read books or magazines. Some knit, work on scrapbooking or even do the ironing! Are there pleasurable things you could do instead of watching TV, such as go for a walk? Substituting pleasurable activities helps to break the vicious cycle I have described above.

It is very important to realize that as you lose weight, you will feel better not only physically but also psychologically—being successful will improve your self-esteem. Feeling better about how you look is the best reinforcement for holding back on red-light choices. As you start to experience success in weight reduction—and we are talking here about permanent weight reduction—you start to consider yourself successful. Successful people hold their bodies differently and interact with people differently. As one reader wrote: "I no longer hide behind a tree every time a camera comes out." As you grow more confident you may feel safe enough to come out into the world. Let people compliment you.

Let me stress again the need to find substitute activities. This is an important tool for breaking bad eating habits. Make a substitute-activities list and use it until you feel sure that your new behaviours and eating patterns are your new habits. Don't beat up on yourself if you slip—it happens to all of us—just get back on the wagon. Having the guts and determination to do this program takes courage. So pat yourself on the back and get on with the journey.

I have been stressing immediate substitute activities but it may also be helpful to think about long-term goals. Have you always had a secret dream or goal—always wanted to take dance lessons, be a tango star or belly dancer, or learn to ski? If you've avoided those dreams because of your self-esteem or body image, maybe now is the time to say this could be possible. Keep that long-term goal in mind when you reach for that red-light food; will that snack help you get on the dance floor?

A cardiologist friend of ours, who is struggling with some bad food habits and poor food choices, wears a plastic bracelet on his left wrist. When he makes a wrong choice he switches the bracelet to his right wrist. This reminds him every time he reaches for something to eat that he has already made one poor choice that day already. He says it's worked for him, so try it if you want a visual aid to help remind you to break bad eating habits. If you do, Rick would be interested in getting your feedback to share with others.

Finally, I encourage you to plan a reward for each week of success on the program—go to a show, buy some flowers, have a long scented bath. Don't buy the new wardrobe yet—that is for later. Remember, be good to yourself.

—Ruth Gallop

E-CLINIC DIARIES

Ruth's comments elicited a great deal of self-recognition among the clinic participants. See if you can hear yourself in their comments:

Ruth's comments really hit home . . . [they] couldn't have come at a better time. I can now get back on track and spend more time reading and studying the red, yellow and green lists of food. I will write down what some of them mean to me and see how many are bringing back childhood memories that I can work on, good or bad. —Casey

When I make bad food choices I feel bad and I want a lift. When I make good food choices I want a reward and guess what that is? Food, in both cases. So I am going to ponder that a bit. I think when I make bad food choices I am going to reread one of your letters or your book, and I am going to make a list of non-food rewards I can have for making good food choices. —Shannon

I think you must have been peeking in my window before I started eating the G.I. way! I know that I am, or have been, an emotional eater and a sneaky eater. As I've said in another letter, I always feel like I'm thinking about what

I can put in my mouth. Of course, I'm still struggling with this and finding ways to change this behaviour . . .

I know I have done many of the things that Ruth talks about. I am guilty of grazing, eating for any emotion and also eating when I'm lonely or bored. One habit Ruth didn't mention that I struggle with is eating to avoid doing a task I don't want to do. I also used to keep snacks at my desk at school and eat too much too often . . .

My worst times for wanting to eat are late afternoon and evenings if I watch TV. I get a very strong urge to have something, preferably something sweet or salty and crunchy. I am trying to stop these high-risk behaviours by drinking a nice hot cup of decaf tea and sometimes having a sugar-free candy. Another way I try to stop this is to wait and tell myself that this feeling will pass. If it just won't pass, then I have a very small green-light snack and have a drink of water to feel fuller. I also find that going and doing something else will take my mind off wanting to eat. The TV watching is my worst enemy! Thank goodness I don't watch much TV. But I do need to learn how to watch it without having the feeling that I need something to eat. I'm still determined and will continue this journey and I will be successful! —Trish

I am really trying to get at the nub of my emotional-eating habits because I think those underlying issues lie at the heart of my problem. Your wife's article gave me food for thought. My mother, a child of the Great Depression, always insisted on our eating everything on our plates and would never waste the smallest of scraps. As much as I fight it, I am the same with my kids. I never explored the possibility of it being tied to her love and approval because I felt much loved in other ways, but perhaps it was. I do know that when I overeat, I force myself to finish the WHOLE ice cream container or the WHOLE bag of cookies to the point where I'm sickened, both in mind and body. Then I indulge in a lot of self-hatred, which leads me to overeat once again. This will take a lot of introspection because I think there are other issues at play as well, but it could be a start of being more self-aware, which, as your wife says, is the first step. —Kate

In the next week, we find out how friends and family can be very important support mechanisms when it comes to avoiding self-sabotage and maintaining motivation.

For Week 6, please see optional meal plan B on pages 177–180 in Part 4.

Week 6 Weight: _____

Week 6 Waist: _____

WEEK 6 DIARY

_____

_____

_____

_____

_____

_____

_____

_____

_____

_____

_____

_____

_____

Week 7
Family and Friends

We are now at the halfway point in the clinic program and you should take a brief timeout to review your progress. First, look at your weight loss over the past six weeks. You should on average have lost a pound a week during this time. There is no yardstick for measuring inches lost around your waist but it should be commensurate with the degree of weight loss (i.e., if you have lost 5 percent of your body weight, your waist measurement should record a similar 5 percent reduction). Second, check that you have indeed cleared out all the red-light foods from your pantry. It's amazing how many things get tucked away at the back! Third, go back through the checklist of behaviour changes, including the emotional ones, to see which ones apply to you and what you are doing about them.

Having a supportive spouse/partner is vital in a successful weight-loss program. It helps to have your own cheering section rather than someone who is running interference and undermining your best efforts. And if you are the one who does most of the cooking, having a supportive partner means you will not have to prepare separate meals—which means there are fewer red-light temptations to deal with.

Both men and women suffer from middle-age spread; look around to see how many men over fifty have "beer bellies." Men under fifty are more at risk from heart disease and stroke than women—but the sexes are equally at risk after this age. Men and women are equally vulnerable to diabetes, and prostate cancer is as prevalent for men as breast cancer is for women. If either or both of you are experiencing weight issues, then it is important that you support each other. If you want to grow old together, then the sooner you adopt the green-light way of eating, the better.

I am writing this testimonial on behalf of my mother who is seventy-nine years young and very grateful for your book. She was diagnosed with diabetes last spring. Her blood sugar count was at 12! and she was a candidate for a heart attack. She was very discouraged and worried. Her doctor gave her six months to do something about it through diet and exercise before putting her on insulin. He prescribed your book and regime and wished her luck.

She was so afraid of having to take insulin every day that she was really motivated to follow your recommendations. She did so faithfully and has lost 23 pounds! More important, her blood sugar has gone down to 4.0. It took nine months. She is not in the danger zone and will not have to take insulin, provided, of course, she continues to eat as she has, following the G.I. Diet. Her doctor is totally amazed at how well she has done. She not only eats as you recommend, but she also exercises on a daily basis. She is completely convinced of the value of your program and tells everyone about it. (You might want to consider hiring her on as a spokesperson, ha ha!) —Monique

Men experience their own version of menopause known as andropause. Andropause results from a drop in testosterone levels. It's testosterone that gives men their male characteristics, both physical and attitudinal, in the same way estrogen gives the female form to women. However, during andropause men's testosterone levels do not fall off as precipitously as do women's estrogen levels during menopause, and generally andropause occurs a few years later than with menopause. (Okay, I know it's not fair, but I didn't write the script!) The reduction in testosterone leads to a slowing metabolism and, along with aging, men experience the same weight-gain issues.

Worse, men are naturally an "apple" shape, versus women's "pear" shape (morphing into "apple" post menopause), which means men carry their excess weight around their waists. Andropause simply accelerates that belly fat accumulation. Unfortunately, carrying fat around your waist is highly detrimental to health. The "beer belly" acts very much like a tumour, feeding the body with a dangerous combination of free fatty acids and proteins, which promote out-of-control cell growth associated with malignant cancers; causes inflammation of the arteries, leading to heart disease and stroke; and increases insulin resistance. If your waist measurement is 37 inches or more (40 inches or more for men), your health is at serious risk.

If your spouse/partner needs to lose weight but appears hesitant about getting onside, here are three approaches that could be persuasive:

- **First: Logic.** You are overweight and that is damaging your health. We can help each other live longer and healthier lives.
- **Second: Blackmail.** Your spouse, children and grandchildren will suffer when you are crippled or die prematurely from diabetes, a heart attack or cancer. How could you abandon us!

- **Third: Stealth.** If all else fails, just change to green-light foods without saying anything. One reader wrote that she did this and the only thing her husband noticed was that his pants were falling down!

Even if your partner is not overweight, he or she will benefit from eating a healthy diet, as many diseases connected with obesity are also associated with diet. All the principal medical and nutritional authorities agree that a diet rich in fruits, vegetables, whole grains, unsaturated fats and lean protein is essential for good health and a longer life—an approach you already know as the G.I. Diet! If weight is not an issue, simply adjust serving sizes and introduce some yellow-light foods. Getting your spouse/partner onside is clearly important and well worth the investment.

With regards to family, eating the green-light way is an excellent choice for the whole family regardless of age. With its emphasis on fruits, vegetables, whole grains, pasta and low-fat dairy products, everybody is getting a healthy well-balanced nutritional diet. Obviously, portion sizes can be adjusted, particularly for youngsters who need those extra calories for growth and activity, as well as for those family members who don't have a weight issue. Children may take a little while adjusting but adjust they will. Remember that you are a role model for your children. Adult children are normally very supportive of their mother in particular trying to improve her health, and how she looks and feels.

Friends, and I include co-workers here as well, can be a curse or a blessing—often a combination of the two. In an e-clinic, Pat was upset by the unhelpful attitude of some of her friends. Here is the response that I wrote to her at the time:

There is no magic to dealing with friends who appear to want to lead you astray. You simply have to tell them that "no" means "no" and that you would appreciate your real friends helping you achieve your goals, rather than making it more difficult. You probably only have to say this once, and if you upset one or two people, then it is worth asking whether they are in fact your real friends . . . in addition you should look to your friends' motivation. If your friends are overweight and see that you are being successful, then they may feel threatened. At least you would know where they are coming from and it may be their own insecurities that are the issue here.

While you have some control over who are your friends, coworkers are another thing. Few of us can control whom we have to work with, and office politics can play havoc with personal relationships. We've all dealt with office gifts of boxes of chocolates, birthday cakes, the "go on, be a devil" office celebratory lunches. Here is what Joan had to say about this:

I've spent many years working through an eating disorder . . . I learned that my abusing food was not different from an alcoholic's abusing alcohol. Food just happened to be the substance that I chose to abuse, to use so I didn't have to feel my feelings. I was such a "good girl" who wouldn't be a drunk, and drugs weren't really available in those days. I couldn't hang out with my old "eating buddies" any more than a drunk getting sober can hang out with his old drinking buddies. I had to find new friends who wanted me to succeed at becoming healthy.

I determine who my friends are by remembering this example: someone I love has a serious drinking or drug problem that is destroying his or her life. He/she goes into treatment or Alcoholics Anonymous, and is attempting to stay sober. As a friend, do I give her/him a bottle of liquor for their birthday or offer them a nice, cold beer on a hot day, telling them that "just one drink" won't hurt them. No, as a friend I want what is best for them, telling them I was so proud of them and letting them know that I am here to help them remain sober.

People are dying from diseases caused by obesity, but food doesn't get the same rap as alcohol or drugs. I cannot change the world's views on eating, but I can change my own. If need be, I am open about my story of my eating disorder to let the person know that food is a serious issue with me. If after they know me and my history, they still push foods on me, I've had to get them out of my life. I can't take the gamble that sometime they'll push food on me when I'm in a bad place and I might just say "Ok, just for this time."

Out of envy or insecurity, many people cannot stand others being successful—and delight in undermining their progress. Sometimes this is called the "tall poppy" syndrome where everyone has to be cut down to the same level.

There are no easy answers except to be upfront about what you are doing: changing the way you eat and why. Ask for their support and, who knows, you may become, as one reader told me, the diet guru of the office, where co-workers, impressed with your success, come to be coached.

And a final word from Karen:

I've also learned that I share my home and office with "diet assassins." I think they think if they can get me to cheat, it absolves their bad eating habits. Last night I found myself making chocolate chip cookies because my husband and co-workers requested them because "[mine] are the best ever." As I was dropping the dough onto the cookie sheet I had an epiphany. I told my husband he could bake as many as he wanted and I wrapped up the rest of the raw dough and brought it to my co-workers with baking instructions. YOU GO GIRL!

E-CLINIC DIARIES

Having your partner, family and friends as cheerleaders—or better still partici-pants—in your green-light journey will help you immeasurably. It's never too soon to start bringing them onside.

My husband has been very supportive throughout this whole process . . . I asked him if he would read the G.I. Diet book so that we could discuss what I was doing, and he has not only read that book . . . but now he has also read Living the G.I. Diet *book.*

Although he has no weight to lose, he has started to change some of his bad eating habits. He ate about 2 to 4 ounces of cheese in his lunch every day and I was worried about the amount of saturated fats he was consuming. Now that he has read your books, he has started to take kidney beans in place of cheese. He has also cut down the amount of sugar and chocolate he used to eat. If he does have some treat, he doesn't eat it in front of me . . . He is very interested in the G.I. Diet and wants to maintain his good health. He also has a family history of diabetes so he wants to dodge the diabetes bullet as much as I do. We are thankful for the knowledge that your books have taught us to help us live a healthier life. We really enjoy all the green-light recipes we have tried from your books and I rarely make anything else for the others in my family. Everyone else in my family is also encouraging me to succeed.

. . . My friends have all been very supportive as well, and they encourage me and want to know how I'm doing. If we do eat out or eat at a friend's

house, they always ask what I can have or ask at what restaurant I could find the right kind of food. I'm very lucky to have so much support from family and friends. —Trish

As far as spousal support is concerned, my husband is all for me losing weight, is willing to try new green-light foods, but will not give up his snacks—the occasional bags of chips, the daily cookies, etc. I can live with that and just make sure I have some acceptable baked goods at the ready for me. —Kate

Well, Rick, I can honestly say I've been on lots of different weight-loss plans and have never had the success that I've had on your G.I. Diet. One thing that I've found out is how helpful it is to have a buddy system. My friend went on your program last March and has lost over 80 pounds, so I get all the tips and advice I need when thing don't seem to go the way I want them to. I just told her I stayed the same weight for two weeks in a row and my measurements aren't changing, but she assured me that things will start to happen. She is right; this week I lost 3 pounds. I've only lost 2 ½ inches since I started, but she once again encouraged me not to get too discouraged because one of these times I will measure myself and find out I've dropped a few inches in a week's time. I know if I keep losing weight then I will have to start losing inches . . . Thank you so much for your help repairing my health. —Casey

In regards to the people who wrote about difficulties with spouses not on the program: I would rather my husband eat exactly what he wants than to have him be focused or engaged in what I am trying to do. His health needs and concerns are different than mine. I know that as he eats bread or granola or whatever really, I am making the choices for me that I need to if I want to reverse the direction of my own health . . . But I feel so good to be in control of my eating—that I feel no need to be in control of my husband's. I want him to enjoy what he enjoys and I want him to respect what I am doing (which he does). —Gail

One of the major challenges to weight loss is eating outside the home where you have far less control. Week 8 will demonstrate how you still eat out and stay with the program even with the ultimate challenge of fast food.

For Week 7, please see optional meal plan B on pages 177–180 in Part 4.

    Week 7 Weight: _____

    Week 7 Waist: _____

WEEK 7 DIARY

_____

_____

_____

_____

_____

_____

_____

_____

_____

_____

_____

_____

_____

_____

_____

Week 8
Eating Out

Eating away from home presents several challenges. The first obstacle you'll face is that the restaurant or fast-food menu naturally limits your choice of food as well as how it is prepared. This is why it's critical to decide ahead of time where you want to dine. To help, I have listed your best green-light choices for most restaurants, family restaurants and fast-food chains.

The second challenge is social. More often than not, dining out is a social occasion with family and friends or co-workers at lunch. You don't want to be a party pooper by making everyone feel uncomfortable with your dietary concerns. More often than not there is the risk of fellow diners egging you to "live a little," which usually means poor food choices, extra drinks and decadent desserts! While there is no easy solution, honesty is the best policy. Be upfront that you have a weight problem that's affecting your health and you would like your family and friends to help you reach your weight goals. No need to ram your diet down the throats of others, but be clear in asking for their support.

Four years ago I was diagnosed as Type II diabetic. I tipped the scale at 400 pounds and was a total mess. I was not able to move, my body ached and I was so miserable I didn't have the will to live. At the obesity clinic they recommended your book. I bought it and decided the G.I. Diet was something I could live with. I started one meal at a time.

Today, I weigh 200 pounds and feel so much better. I can't begin to thank you for all the wonderful ideas you have put into your books. I have been on every diet known to man. I have had my stomach stapled and have done everything I could have done to lose the weight I needed to lose. Nothing I did worked until I read your books. They are direct, straightforward and to the point. The red, yellow and green are wonderful because anyone can follow that even if you are colour-blind. Many, many thanks. —Marie

FAST FOOD

Most of the leading fast-food restaurants have introduced menu items that are lower in fat and calories. However, a word of warning, when reducing fat levels companies may well boost sugar and sodium (salt) levels to offset any perceived loss of flavour. Remember, salt retains liquid, which is the last thing you need when you're trying to lose weight, yet alone trying to keep your blood pressure down. If you are not sure about salt levels, ask your server for a nutritional information sheet, which most family and fast-food restaurant chains carry.

A few ground rules:

- Always eat burgers and sandwiches opened-faced, throwing away the top slice of bread or bun.
- Use, at most, one-third of the salad dressing normally provided in a sachet, as it contains far more than you would ever need, and adds only unnecessary calories and salt to your meal. Choose light or vinaigrette dressings over creamy ones.
- Chicken is now featured in many fast-food restaurants. Make sure you ask for grilled chicken, not fried (crispy).

Here is a more detailed rundown of your best choices at some of the larger fast-food chains:

Subway

This chain has been a pacesetter in the fast-food industry in reducing fat and calories in its meals. Subway's 6-inch/6-gram-fat subs on whole wheat or honey oat bread are your best choices. Just be careful not to load on those high-fat/-calorie extras such as cheese, bacon and high-sugar sauces. Mr. Sub and other similar sandwich chains are following Subway's lead.

McDonald's

McDonald's grilled chicken salads are a good bet with a low-fat dressings. You can even go for a Fruit 'n' Yogurt Parfait dessert (hold the granola).

Harvey's

Grilled chicken salad/burger or a veggie burger are your best bet.

Burger King

Unfortunately this chain is one of the few that does not appear to have got the message that people want healthy options. Only the veggie burger (without mayo) and a garden salad makes the grade.

Wendy's

Grilled Chicken Go Wrap is your only alternative though you might consider a large chili with side salad. Wendy's chicken salads are to be avoided as they are high in fat and sodium.

Pizza Hut

Normally I recommend avoiding pizza restaurants, so I am delighted to see that Pizza Hut has made a real effort to improve its offerings. Your best bet is Thin 'N Crispy Pizzas and Fit 'n Delicious Pizzas (2 slices maximum) with garden salads and light dressings.

Taco Bell

Taco Bell's line of Fresco tacos are acceptable green-light choices but are very high in sodium. Steer clear of the rest of the menu except the side salads.

KFC

Until KFC adopts grilled, as opposed to fried, chicken as they have in the United States, it's a place to avoid.

RESTAURANTS

As it's impossible to list restaurants by name, I've provided a quick rundown of different types of restaurants instead.

Family Restaurants

This is a fast-growing segment of the restaurant business and offers a very wide choice of foods and good value for a family eating out.

Though there are a few national chains, such as Swiss Chalet or Kelsey's, most are local operations, making it impossible to analyze individual restaurants in the space available.

However, the one overriding caution with these restaurants is portion size. Many serving sizes are large enough for two people. On a recent road trip, my wife and I found we could split many, if not most, of the courses and still come away satisfied.

If you are watchful, you can easily find many green-light alternatives to suit the entire family.

All-You-Can-Eat Buffets

This can be your worst or best option depending on your level of self-control. Best to do a quick reconnaissance of the whole buffet before you start to fill your plate. This way you can pick out your best green-light choices ahead of time.

Italian

Start with a good bean and vegetable soup such as minestrone. Avoid cream-based soups. For the main course your best option is grilled, roasted or braised fish, chicken or veal. You may order pasta as a side dish if you wish, though you would be better off with an extra serving of vegetables.

Greek

Grilled or baked seafood is an excellent choice as is the classic chicken souvlaki. Just watch your serving sizes. Instead of the potatoes, which are frequently served along with rice, order double vegetables. You must ask for both your salad dressing and feta to be served on the side so you can control your servings.

Chinese

This type of food can present some real challenges. Much of the food is deep-fried with sweet sauces. Sodium levels are usually astronomic and the rice is glutinous and red-light (short-grain rice has a much higher G.I. than long-grain rice such as basmati). Though you can make do with steamed or stir-fried vegetables, this kind of restaurant would be my last resort when eating out.

Indian/South Asian

This is one of your best restaurant choices because of the cuisine's focus on vegetables, legumes and long-grain rice. Servings of meat, poultry or fish tend to be modest. However, make sure that food is not fried, particularly not in "ghee" (clarified butter), which is a highly saturated fat. Also be cautious with all creamy sauces and side dishes such as mangoes/papayas, raisins and coconut slices as they have a higher G.I. and can pack a lot of calories if you aren't careful.

Mexican/Latin American

Tex-Mex dishes can be heavy on cheese, refried beans and sour cream, which are all red-light. Your best bet is to look for grilled seafood, chicken or meat, as well as dishes made with beans (not refried). Vegetable-based soups such as gazpacho are an excellent choice.

Thai

Thai restaurants tend to be heavy on red-light sauces, often using full-fat coconut milk. Here it's best to stick with a starter such as lemongrass soup, green mango salad, or mussels in a lemongrass broth. Follow this with a Thai beef salad or stir-fry with chicken and vegetables. Skip the peanut sauce.

Japanese

This is a good green-light choice once you get beyond the sushi and tempura. Sushi is red-light because of the glutinous rice it is made with. Order the sashimi instead. Watch the quantity of soy sauce, which should be thought of as liquid salt! The beef and vegetable stir-fries and grilled fish are excellent choices. You might try Nabemono, a healthy fondue with broth rather than oil as the cooking medium.

If you are dining in a group you might not have any say as to the choice of restaurant. In that case, a little planning and some careful choices can help you over the hurdles:

TOP TEN DINING TIPS

1. If possible, just before you go out, have a small bowl of high-fibre, green-light cold cereal (such as All-Bran) with skim milk and sweetener. I often add a couple of spoonfuls of no-fat/no-sugar fruit yogurt. This will take the edge off your appetite and get some fibre into your digestive system, which will help reduce the G.I. of your upcoming meal.

2. Once seated in the restaurant, drink a glass of water. It will help you feel fuller.

3. Remember to eat slowly to allow your brain the time it needs to realize you are full. Put your fork down between mouthfuls and savour your meal.

4. Once the basket of rolls or bread—which you will ignore—has been passed around the table, ask the server to remove it. The longer it sits, the more tempted you will be to dig in.

5. Order a soup or salad first and tell the server you would like this as soon as possible. This will keep you from sitting there hungry while others are filling up on bread. For soups, go for vegetable or bean-based, the chunkier the better. Avoid any that are cream-based, such as vichyssoise. For salads, keep the dressing on the side. Then you can use a fraction of what the restaurant would normally pour over your greens. Avoid Caesar salads, which come pre-dressed and often pack as many calories as a burger.

6. Since you probably won't get boiled new potatoes and can't be sure of what kind of rice is being served, ask for a double serving of vegetables instead. I have yet to find a restaurant that won't oblige.

7. Stick with low-fat cuts of meat or poultry. If necessary, you can remove the skin. Duck is usually too high in fat. Fish and shellfish are excellent choices but shouldn't be breaded, battered or fried. Tempura is more fat and flour than filling. Remember that servings tend to be generous in restaurants, so eat only 4 to 6 ounces (the size of a pack of cards) and leave the rest. Entree sharing is also a popular option.

8. As with salads, ask for any sauces to be served on the side.

9. For dessert, fresh fruit and berries—without the ice cream—are your best choice. Most other desserts are a dietary disaster. My advice to you is to avoid dessert. If a birthday cake is being passed around, share your piece with someone. A couple of forkfuls with your coffee should get you off the hook with minimal dietary damage!

10. Order only decaffeinated coffee. Skim-milk decaf cappuccino is our family's favorite choice.

E-CLINIC DIARIES

Eating out always generates a great deal of discussion. I was delighted to see that most clinic members were up to the challenge and coping admirably.

"Waste not, want not" is a mindset that has been totally embedded in me. This is one of my problems right now with food. I just cannot go to a buffet or anywhere where there is lots of food because it is too overwhelming to see all that food and not try it. Portions are critical because if I put a large amount on my plate, I have difficulty throwing any away. —Chandra

While it is easy to plan lots of veggies, etc., while at home, and avoid red/ yellow–light foods, it is sometimes more difficult to do so when dining out. Though I have not been perfect in this regard, I do know that I have made far better choices than I would if I were not on this program . . . I do not have staggering weight loss, but I am happy to see the numbers on the scale moving down, not up, particularly at a time of year when I find I am more sedentary. —Linda

What amazes me at this stage of the clinic is the difference in my feelings about eating in general and eating out. I'm very pleased that this [G.I. Diet] way of eating has started to become second nature to me. We ate out this weekend at a buffet-style restaurant and it was just natural for me to choose the correct foods without any anxiety about things I should not choose. I actually didn't even want to choose those things. And I even felt badly watching some other people at the restaurant who were very overweight eating huge amounts of all the wrong foods. When I saw one woman filling her plate with small servings of green-light foods, I wanted to tap her on the shoulder and ask if she was in this clinic, too! She was a small size, so this is probably how she eats every day. —Trish

I was proud of myself this week. We had to go to Alabama, and those people know how to cook good-tasting food. Unfortunately, it's all unhealthy, loaded with bacon grease for seasoning, fried foods, etc. I had smartened up though and took my apples, pears, carrots, radishes and protein drinks for breakfast. I would eat with them, but very small portions of only the healthiest foods on the table and fill up on the other stuff. Every time I had to stop at McDonald's for my wife, I ate out of the ice chest. I still don't have her on board and probably never will. She does ok part of the time, but the other 60 percent she wants to eat the "comfort" foods of the South and sweets. The weight isn't tumbling off me at a fast rate, but I feel stronger and better. I can really tell a difference in my clothes. My belt has gone from the last hole to the first and it's still loose at that. I plan to start working more exercise and walking into my schedule. —Howard

I think one of my saving graces is the 10 percent wiggle room and your advice to savour the cheat if we are going that route. I don't think I cheat every day but have to tell you yesterday I was at one of the warehouse stores where samples were provided. They were sampling the mini cream puffs. The sample sizes were half of the normal puff. I just had to have one!!! But I ate it as slowly as I could—delicious—and that was it for the day. —Barbara

Interesting week—I've been at a resort and I thought I was a goner when they delivered warm cinnamon buns to the room the first morning. But I have managed to make fairly good choices most of the time, I think. Eating in restaurants was a bit of a challenge. You have to mine the menu for something green-light to eat. I found the less expensive the restaurant, the harder it was. —Shannon

Eating out will always be a challenge, but with the above information you should be able to make the best of a potentially difficult situation. In Week 9 we will deal with two of the biggest frustrations in losing weight: reaching a plateau and falling off the wagon.

For Week 8, please see optional meal plan B on pages 177–180 in Part 4.

Week 8 Weight: _____

Week 8 Waist: _____

WEEK 8 DIARY

_____

_____

_____

_____

_____

Week 9
Staying the Course

By the end of the first two months of the program, two issues preoccupied many of the e-clinic participants, as evidenced in their diaries: reaching a weight-loss plateau and falling off the wagon. These are perhaps the most frustrating challenges that people on any diet experience. Let me give you a sense of why these challenges present themselves and suggest some strategies for coping with them.

REACHING A PLATEAU

After diligently eating the green-light way and losing weight steadily for successive weeks, it is difficult to accept that a break in the pattern, unfair as it may be, is inevitable. Weight loss never occurs in a straight line, but always in a series of steps or plateaus.

There are a couple of principal causes. First, hormonal shifts triggered by a woman's monthly cycle or menopause cause the body to retain fluid (for example, if you usually wear rings they might feel tight on your fingers). This is nearly always a temporary state. As your hormones shift back to their previous levels, so will your fluids.

The second most common cause is "portion creep," because a weight-loss plateau can occur when you have let your guard down and allowed your portion or serving size to increase. This is easy to do as you have watched the pounds steadily drop off; not surprisingly, complacency can set in. A useful tool in keeping you on track is dividing your place into three sections (see page 24): half the plate should consist of at least two vegetables; one-quarter should consist of a protein (meat, fish, chicken or tofu); and the remaining quarter can consist of rice, potatoes or pasta. Remember to use small lunch-sized plates instead of oversized dinner plates.

Since hormonal shifts and complacency can cause your weight to fluctuate significantly from day to day, I suggest you restrict your weigh-in to once a week. Then you can avoid the disappointment of the short-term aberrations and focus on your long-term success. One reader wrote to me and said that she had become very frustrated with the daily variations in weight and decided to weigh herself once a month.

She said there was not a single month in the past eighteen months when she had not lost some weight, and her frustration level had dropped significantly.

I'm sure you hear this all the time, but thank you for writing your book. Without question it has saved my life. I've been overweight my whole life. I have tried every diet known to man. I've been a Type II diabetic for fourteen years. I was up to three diabetic medications twice daily with high blood pressure. I would love to be able to tell you what I weighed, but household scales would not weigh me. My doctor said that without drastic changes I could be on insulin within six months. I bought your book the next day and read it from cover to cover. Everything was so clear and easy to follow. On your inside cover you had a testimonial from Derek that said he lost 85 pounds in twenty-two weeks. That amazed me, so I figured if he could do it, so could I. After six weeks I could finally weigh myself on my scale at home: 370 pounds. Now, thirteen weeks later I weigh 315 pounds. That's nineteen weeks and my doctor estimates close to 90 pounds; I've gone from a waist of 56 inches to 46 inches. I have a long way to go but I am sure I can live the G.I. way the rest of my life. I'm going to become a grandfather for the first time in a few weeks. Thank you for making it possible for me to see my granddaughter grow up. —Lee

When playing the averages, patience is a virtue! Just keep on the green-light track and the weight will continue to come off. Some clinic participants also wondered why they sometimes seem to be losing inches but not pounds, and sometimes pounds but not inches. Remember, everyone is different, and weight loss doesn't ever happen in a straight line; eventually both the inches and pounds will come off—guaranteed!

Don't let an irregularity on the scale get you down, although nothing is quite as frustrating as hitting a weight-loss plateau. But if you hang in there and don't use food to console yourself, you will reach your weight-loss target.

FALLING OFF THE WAGON

Like a weight-loss plateau, falling off the wagon is bound to happen sooner or later. And while I don't encourage it, it's acceptable as long as it's the exception and not the rule. The diet isn't meant to be a straitjacket, after all. If you do your best to eat the green-light way 90 percent of the time, you will still lose weight. The odd lapse, at worst, will delay you by a week or two from reaching your target weight. So don't be too hard on yourself; just get right back on the plan with the next meal. Some people make the mistake of feeling so bad about having a slip-up that they just give up. But you should anticipate that you will fall off the wagon from time to time. The best way to handle it is to learn why it happened and decide how you will handle the situation the next time. By now you have the knowledge and tools to do just that.

Although most people find that their cravings diminish after a few weeks on the G.I. Diet, because of the levelling effects green-light eating has on blood sugar levels, there will be times when a craving will surface. Here's how to handle the situation:

1. Distract yourself with an activity. Call a friend, fold a basket of laundry, take out the garbage or go for a walk. Sometimes a craving will pass.

2. If you are still have the craving, pinpoint the flavour that you want and find a green-light food that has it. For example, if you want something sweet and creamy, try low-fat yogurt or ice cream with no added sugar. If you want something salty, have a couple of olives or a dill pickle, or some hummus with veggies. If it's chocolate you crave, try half a chocolate-flavoured nutrition bar or a mug of instant light hot chocolate. There are many green-light versions of the foods we normally reach for when a craving strikes.

3. Sometimes nothing but a piece of chocolate or a spoonful of peanut butter will do. If this is the case, have a small portion and really enjoy it. Eat it slowly and savour the experience. Chalk it up to that 10 percent leeway you're allowed on the G.I Diet. Just make sure you're staying green-light 90 percent of the time.

Remember, the 10 percent "wiggle room" I mentioned earlier gives you permission to enjoy that extra serving or occasional drink. It is meant to help you stay with the program, so use it wisely.

E-CLINIC DIARIES

If you really want to make a permanent change in the way you eat and look, keep planning ahead—especially if you've hit a plateau or find yourself repeatedly falling off the wagon. Think about where you might have slipped back, consciously or unconsciously, into your old food habits. Here is what some of our e-clinic members had to say about their frustrations and successes:

I will be going to my doctor next week . . . I should be down at least 11 pounds since I last saw him . . . Although my waist measurement hasn't gone down that significantly, my pants are fitting so much better and looser . . . My friend Ingrid has lost 14 pounds (she went on this program with me). She is beyond thrilled and ecstatic and says she FEELS great and so much better than she used to. She thought she would never see weight loss again and is very grateful. THANKS from the bottom, sides and tops of both our hearts. —Shirley

To help stay away from being too long on the plateau I try to do the following things:

1. Plan, shop, and prepare green-light meals and snacks. This helps keep the stress of finding things to eat at a minimum and makes the whole journey more pleasurable.

2. I try to keep my portion sizes smaller. I like the term "portion creep" that you used. It definitely is something that I have to continually keep in mind.

3. I find that I have to eat less at night. I know it's not pleasant to go to bed hungry, but if I feel somewhat hungry at night it seems that I have a much better chance of losing some weight. I don't mean being ravenous.

4. I have to make sure that I move more. It's very comfortable to hibernate in the cold of winter but I do feel much more energetic if I do some exercises that get my blood pumping and my metabolism working harder. I have to go easy on this because of my arthritis and fibromyalgia so that I don't get too much pain, but it helps to exercise regularly and gently.

5. My worst nemesis is sitting in front of the TV. That's when I often have the feeling that I have to have something, anything. Some days I feel like I'm prowling around trying to satisfy some urgent need. I'm still trying to change my mindset on this problem, and getting out of the house and of course turning off the TV are helpful but I'm also working on just relaxing in front of the TV and not feeling this old habit. Conquering this will definitely help me stay off the plateaus.

I will continue to persevere and try to be patient with my journey on the green-light highway. I feel proud of myself for what I have accomplished so far and I look forward to more successes. —Trish

I am happy that the scale is moving downward, although slower than some people are finding, but making some progress and seeing these results are personally encouraging. Some are having great success and their stories are certainly encouraging! Others are more like me in their "slow and steady wins the race," and I think that just seeing that scale moving downward, even though it is slower than some, reminds me that I didn't put on the weight in a matter of weeks. . . . as long as it is "leaving" bit by bit, I am happy . . . plus, I am sure that my blood chemistry will show improvement, and that is my main concern. I did have a few people comment on the fact that I must have lost some weight, so that also is encouraging. —Linda*

Week 9, I can't believe it. Where have the weeks gone? I am disappointed I didn't lose any inches this week but am happy nonetheless. My clothes are fitting better and this week I was able to wear a couple of tops that I had pulled out the back of the closest. That was a great feeling. —Barbara*

I have a doctor's appointment soon—my annual checkup—and I know he will be taking blood tests that will include the A1C level. The last visit I had was just before starting the clinic and my A1C at that time was 8.4. I am anxious to see what it will be this time. I know my doctor will be pleased to see I have lost weight (19 pounds so far). At the last office visit, he wanted to put me on an additional oral medication along with the Metformin that I already take. I don't think that will be necessary now. —Joanne*

When I was accepted into the clinic I had serious doubts about staying with it . . . I was ready to quit before I even got started! Well . . . I dove in, and must say the recipes were great. I made a few soups, and the scones, the oat cakes, three kinds of muffins and bean-based brownies. I had no room left in my freezers! I set up an "eat every 2 ½ hour" schedule for myself, and I think it was less than three days when I noticed it . . . I wasn't hungry anymore; the cravings were gone. It was liberating, I actually had to watch the clock to make sure I didn't miss a meal or snack . . . I was away from home for four days and ate in restaurants, and still lost a pound. I go out for lunch with the girls and am still losing. I just make smarter choices. I never feel like I am missing out on something. And yes . . . I use the 10 percent wiggle room (which on occasion has been more like 20 percent!), but every meal I am home for is total green-light . . .

    I am sure my weight loss will slow down even more in the future, but my goal is to lose 1 pound a week until a year is up, I feel I will level off when my body is happy with the end result. I really wish I'd done this years ago. I wasted time being obsessed with my weight and body image. All in all, I have lost my 10 percent (+ more) that I wanted to lose, 6.5 inches from my waist, and my blood sugar is down even with dropping most of my meds. I stopped taking glyburide after my first four weeks, and have now gone to two Metformin a day from four. —Ade*

Even though my weight and waist have not drastically reduced, I can certainly feel a difference in my clothes. I no longer have to lie down on the bed to zip my jeans . . . ha ha! It is such a motivator to have wiggle room in my clothes, so I feel like the Energizer Bunny . . . This will be a lifetime of eating and living better. Thank you, Rick! —Chandra*

Underlying all we have discussed about plateauing and falling off the wagon is the importance of staying motivated. If you sense you are wavering, reread Week 5 on the importance of motivation. Without it you are unlikely to stay the course—and that goes double when you're entertaining and during holidays when red-light foods are literally surrounding you! Week 10 offers strategies for coping with these celebratory times when diets often get thrown out the window, and will help keep you on track as you slim down.

For Week 9, please see optional meal plan B on pages 177–180 in Part 4.

    Week 9 Weight: _____

      Week 9 Waist: _____

WEEK 9 DIARY

_____

_____

_____

_____

_____

_____

_____

_____

_____

_____

_____

_____

_____

_____

_____

_____

_____

_____

_____

_____

Week 10
Celebrations: Holidays and Entertaining

Food and celebrations are inextricably intertwined. Since earliest recorded times, food and drink have been central when people get together for social or celebratory reasons. Whether they're events driven by the calendar—such as Thanksgiving, Christmas, New Year's—or family affairs such as anniversaries, birthdays, weddings or barbecues—all have one thing in common, food and drink—usually lots of it and usually the red-light sort! However, it really is not that hard not only to survive, but also enjoy and eat well at these gatherings.

If you are worried that people will be watching what you eat, always keep some green-light food on your plate, and nibble very slowly. Don't assume the skinny people are having loads of fun—they could be as worried as or more worried about the food than you! Remember, as you lose weight, people may comment—usually positively. Thank them for the compliment. If they ask, "Have you lost weight?" Just answer, "Yes, I have. Thanks for noticing," and move on. No need for detailed explanations.

ENTERTAINING AT HOME

When you are entertaining friends or family at a cocktail party or buffet you can control the kind of food that is served. Nibbles and snacks can all be green-light. For example, serve hummus or salsa with raw vegetables and smoked salmon on cucumber. Meats can be lean deli meats with assorted mustards. Make rice salads such as the Waldorf Chicken and Rice Salad on page 218. Put out fruit platters with flavoured yogurt dips. Serve decaf coffee with our homemade Cran-Apple Oatmeal Bars (see page 268) and fresh berries.

If you are cooking a meal for your family other than the traditional holiday ones mentioned above, try some of the recipes mentioned in Part 4, or check out the *The G.I. Diet Cookbook* for more delicious entertaining suggestions.

THE CELEBRATORY FAMILY DINNER

You may be preparing the dinner or attending someone else's. Some of the traditional foods are yellow- or even red-light, but with adjustments you can enjoy many of them.

As an example, we have taken the classic turkey-based dinner normally associated with Thanksgiving and Christmas, but with many components that can be featured any time of the year. This will please even the fussiest relative.

THE CLASSIC TURKEY DINNER

Soup: If you have soup before the turkey, prepare a stock- or broth-based soup. Use fresh herbs and vegetables to flavour the soup, avoiding cream or butter additions.

> *I started the G.I. Diet as a way to control my blood sugars, which were out of control. I have Type II diabetes, and my control was so bad (A1C of 8.7) that my doctor put me on another medication and threatened to put me on insulin. While I lost around 5 pounds, the best result was when I visited my doctor yesterday. My A1C went down to 6.7! My doctor and I were both very pleased. It was due to my change of diet, watching what I eat when we go out, and keeping fruits and vegetables in the house. Thank you for making it so easy!*
> —Susan

The turkey: This is easy. You can prepare a traditional bird and eat the white breast meat—skin off, of course. Make a stuffing using wild or basmati rice, apples or mushrooms, celery, onions and seasoning, leaving out the bread crumbs. Pork loin or even a short leg of lamb, with the fat well trimmed, are other acceptable alternatives.

Cranberry sauce: This can be made from scratch using sucralose (Splenda) to sweeten the cranberries. Add some orange pieces and slivered almonds for a delicious crunch.

Salad: Always serve a large salad with homemade green-light dressing. Try serving this before the main course to help fill you up. Fancy it up with toasted pecans, a sprinkling of dried cranberries, or a scattering of crumbled blue cheese. Ruth makes a simple salad using romaine lettuce, sliced strawberries and a raspberry or balsamic vinaigrette. It's very easy and quite pretty.

Sweet potatoes: If sweet potatoes are an essential part of the feast then go ahead, but instead of using brown sugar, orange juice or maple syrup, try mashing them with some powdered ginger, light non-hydrogenated margarine, pepper and hot water if needed. Or you can try roasted butternut squash with a balsamic vinegar glaze.

Vegetables: For vegetable side dishes, make a colourful dish of steamed vegetables, then lightly sauté in olive oil with seasoning such as thyme, sage, garlic and fresh pepper. This can be a very festive holiday dish if you use red and green peppers and snow peas as the main vegetables.

Dessert: No need to feel cheated when it comes to dessert. Dessert can be an apple or fruit crumble served with fat-free yogurt with sweetener or a fat-free flavoured yogurt sweetened with Splenda. Or use a no-sugar-added low-fat ice cream or frozen yogurt. For an elegant dessert, make a Pavlova with lemon-flavored yogurt cheese and fresh berries.

No one will leave the table feeling hungry! Just remember to fill half of your plate with vegetables, one-quarter with protein, and one-quarter with potatoes or rice. Keep portion sizes in line with G.I Diet requirements and enjoy.

COCKTAIL AND DRINKS PARTIES

It is quite easy to enjoy cocktail parties on the G.I. Diet. Keep a glass in your hand. It can be soda water with a twist of lime; or, if you want alcohol, try one long drink such as a white wine spritzer; or have one glass of red and then switch to soda water. If you don't have something in your hand, someone will pass you a drink you haven't chosen, or your hands will find bowls of food to graze on. Make sure you consume the alcohol with some food to slow the rate at which your body will metabolize it. Try to avoid beer and fancy cocktails, which are caloric nightmares. Look for nibbles that are green-light if possible. Do not station yourself beside the bowls of nuts—they may be green-light but restricting yourself to a small handful may be difficult.

BUFFETS

Buffets can be heaven or hell: heaven in that you usually have a wide choice of foods, which enables you to make better choices; hell because of all the fancy, calorie-laden temptations laid out before you. How many times have you kept loading your plate as you progress down the line, finding yet another delicious temptation that you just have to try? By the end of the line, you're wishing you had a larger plate and you hadn't included, or at least had taken a smaller serving, of some of your earlier choices.

Start with just a salad. This helps fill you up a little and takes the edge off your appetite. Then take a plate—look for a luncheon and not an enormous dinner plate—and focus on vegetables and lean protein.

For dessert, look for fruit platters only. Give all other desserts a miss unless you are absolutely certain they are green-light. Finish up with a decaf coffee or tea.

E-CLINIC DIARIES
Changing eating habits during the holiday season is challenging but key to your success is planning ahead and looking for green-light options.

As I write this, I am sitting at a wonderful seaside resort at which my family and I are celebrating Christmas. It is an all-inclusive holiday, which allows the guests unlimited amounts of food pretty well all day as well as drinks. The ultimate challenge to the GI-er . . . bread and rolls tend to be white, no hot oatmeal for breakfast, desserts galore, cheese plates, pasta bars, long ice cream counters—you get the picture!

Needless to say, it has been very, very difficult to resist the temptations. I do have a supply of raw almonds with me and along with some cold bran cereal and fresh fruit—that's breakfast. I make a sandwich out of lots of raw veggies, egg slices, lean meat and more fruit for lunch. Supper is far more difficult, but I'm trying to eat fish (had catfish last night, but it was fried) and salads. I'm enjoying myself and intend to continue to do so within the confines of my new "lifestyle." —Kate

I overindulged during the season but am back on track this morning. I could give you myriad reasons, but they are standard for everyone, and no one held a fork up to my head and forced me to participate or sample what I was cooking, or eat at holiday socials. A few good things despite my lack of progress are:

1. The food that is not part of my lifestyle change did not taste anything as good as it did the last time I ate it.

2. I am determined not to belittle and degrade myself because I made unwise choices. I am moving on.

3. My body actually can tell the difference in poor eating. I am tired and depleted—my energy has evaporated and I want it back. —Shirley

Our big celebration is on Christmas Eve and we serve some traditional Polish dishes. I handled the whole thing by eating whatever I wanted in small portions. It worked well both with my blood sugar and weight. I am pleased with the whole outcome. It is most likely easy for me to do this as I have never been a big eater but rather a "wrong eater" and years ago I learned to just quit eating when full, not even one more bite. —Sharon

We had our 3 adult children home for the holidays . . . I planned my menus and precooked a lot of food (all green). I ate well—green at all the meals. My major brain failure came in "snacking." I ate peanuts while playing cards, I ate peanut brittle (and lots of it) and all the other "treats." After everyone left yesterday I felt like crying. I was very depressed and unhappy with myself and did a lot of put-downs and name-calling . . . I am still disappointed with myself but I think I need to put it behind me and consider this the first day of the rest of my life . . . I know I can eat in a restaurant and I can have company for meals without falling down. I must do something different about having red snacks sitting out on the table twenty-four hours a day. —Corinne

I feel a bit stuck, but remain positive—mainly because I got through the food frenzy of Christmas without eating any red-light foods. No sugar, bread, cookies, candy. Not even a taste. I feel this is a success in itself. I wish the scales reflected it, but I am determined to pay more attention to how I feel than how much I lost or remained the same. —Gail

Several times when my company arrives for our weekly card games I serve my friends my diet foods and they didn't even know. One friend in particular insists on bringing me the wrong foods. When she said you won't eat any of the cakes, cookies or candy that I bring, yet you serve us the same as these foods at the card games, I smiled and said, "I do eat them, but mine are much healthier! Seeing as you like them so much, I have copied the recipes for you so now you will be able to serve them to me the next time we play cards at your house." Then I made the comment if anyone wants to know who your real friends are, just tell them you are going on a diet. A true friend will try to help. I've lost 3 pounds since last week because I changed my way of eating and went back to the proper G.I. Diet. I'd like the inches to drop off faster but the main thing is I am losing inches, pounds and have perfect blood sugar readings. —Casey

Next week we will be examining in detail why all of you picked up this book in the first place, namely diabetes and your health. Other than your genes, good health is largely determined by what and how much you eat, and is the one thing that you have complete control over.

For Week 10, please see optional meal plan B on pages 177–180 in Part 4.

Week 10 Weight: _____

Week 10 Waist: _____

WEEK 10 DIARY

_____

_____

_____

_____

_____

_____

_____

_____

Week 11
Diabetes and Your Health

As we age we become increasingly prone to life's major diseases. Heart disease, stroke, hypertension, cancer, diabetes and Alzheimer's are all diseases primarily associated with aging. This is demonstrated by health care expenditures in North America that are four to five times higher for those over sixty-five years of age. The following Canadian chart indicates this change in spending as we age.

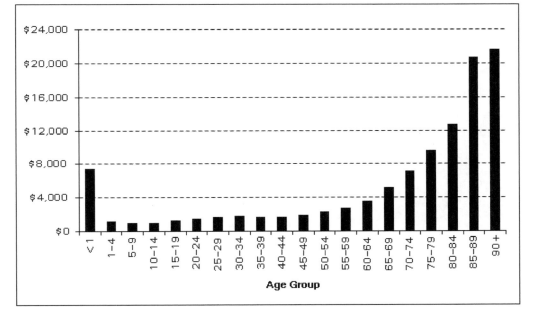

Sources: National Health Expenditure Database, CIHI; Population, Statistics Canada, 2005.

The kind of food you choose to eat—and the resulting impact upon your weight and health—is undoubtedly the single most significant controllable factor in determining whether you are at risk for these killer diseases ("controllable" means those things you can influence, as opposed to factors such as your genes, which you cannot). "You are what you eat" has never been more true.

I am a Type II diabetic, fifty-three years old and about 50 pounds over my ideal weight. My sugar testing in the morning had gone up to 12.7, and I felt dizzy and tired all the time. I knew I had to do something beyond taking the pills. I saw your book and had remembered I was given a G.I brochure when I was diagnosed as a diabetic, read it and tossed it. I started your diet and in one week I dropped my sugar testing to 7.3. I was hooked. I starting baking and cooking everything in the book.

At first I was afraid because when you hear "eating healthy," I remembered what that meant years ago: whole wheat bread that tasted like sand, chicken that was boiled, eating salad until your lips bleed. I didn't want to do that again. But these recipes tasted great and I enjoyed and shared them with my family. You have given me the tools to reduce my sugar level and stop me from becoming a Type I diabetic. My goal is to reduce my sugar level and weight to the point that I will not be a diabetic at all. Thank you.
—Vernon (father of five children and grandfather of two)

Middle age can be a wake-up call to the realization that if you want to live a longer, active life, you need to eat foods that support your health—not damage it—and help you maintain a healthy weight. Do it both for yourself as well as for your family and friends.

ARE YOU AN APPLE OR PEAR?

As you are now aware, there is a strong correlation between obesity and health. What you may not know is that obesity, as traditionally measured by your BMI, is not necessarily the best guide to assessing your health risk. It's where the fat is stored that is the real issue.

The location of that extra fat around the waistline is particularly hazardous for diabetics. It is also associated with other major diseases, as shown in the results of a recently released worldwide survey of 27,000 people carried out by the Population Health Research Institute at McMaster University, which indicated that people who carried their extra weight around their waists were at far greater risk of serious diseases than those who carried their weight lower down on their hips.

Such people are described as "apple shaped," whereas people who carry fat on their hips are called "pear shaped." So it's the apple shaped among us who need to be particularly concerned about their health. This is not to dismiss the relationship between being overweight and therefore at greater risk of disease, but it's a major refinement. From this study came the table below, showing the risk of life-threatening diseases versus weight and waist measurement.

This information is particularly important for women in their menopausal years when the reduction in estrogen levels results in losing the traditional pear-shaped figure. As we discussed at the outset of the program, your body begins to adopt the traditional male apple shape, which as you can see below, is a major predictor of your health risk.

WEIGHT	BMI	WAIST (inches) Women 35" or less Men 40" or less	WAIST (inches) Women 35" plus Men 40" plus
Normal	18.0—24.9	No risk increase	No risk increase
Overweight	25.0—29.9	Increased risk	High risk
Obese	30.0—39.9	High risk	Very high risk

So those of you who have a BMI of 30 or more—a waist measurement of 35 inches or more for women and 40 inches or more for men—are in the Very High Risk category for developing heart disease, stroke, hypertension (high blood pressure) and certain types of cancer—breast, uterine and colon.

A further refinement is your waist-to-hip ratio. This is measured by dividing your hip measurement into your waist measurement. A healthy ratio for women is 0.85 or below, and 0.95 or below for men. So, as a woman, for instance, if your hips measure 48 inches and your waist 44 inches, you waist-to-hip ratio is 0.92, which puts you firmly at risk. Conversely, if your hips were 48 inches but your waist was reduced to 40 inches, your ratio would be an acceptable 0.83.

As discussed, this "beer belly" is not just surplus weight, which would be bad enough, but it acts like a huge tumour in that it boosts hormone levels, which stimulates cell growth, and causes inflammation, leading to clogged arteries. This is not a passive depository of fat; rather, it is a hostile appendage that is actively undermining your health.

DIABETES

The principal outcome of being overweight is diabetes. But the combination of high blood sugar and obesity place the diabetic into the high-risk category for heart disease, stroke, hypertension, loss of vision (retinopathy) and kidney disease. As if that wasn't bad enough, there is new research that clearly demonstrates a direct association between higher A1C levels and lower cognitive function in diabetics.

Fortunately, the G.I. Diet is extremely effective in managing the causes and symptoms of diabetes by helping to regulate blood sugar. I have had thousands of diabetics write that they had been able to reduce, or in some cases—with their doctor's supervision and approval—go off their medication entirely. By reducing your weight and better managing your blood sugar levels with your green-light foods, you have every opportunity to reduce your risk of this dreadful disease. As I have said before, you now have the tools, and you should most certainly have the motivation, given the horrendous health risks associated with diabetes, to do something about it.

Heart disease, stroke and cancer account for approximately ⅔ of all deaths in North America. The G.I. Diet may also be able to help reduce your chances of developing them:

HEART ATTACK AND STROKE

For many years, heart attacks were considered to be a man's domain, which still is more often than not the case for men under the age of fifty, but after that it becomes a common concern for both men and women. The U.S. Archives of Internal Medicine reported that researchers followed 88,000 healthy women for twenty-four years to see how their food choices impacted their risk of heart attack and stroke. Those who ate a diet that emphasized fruits, vegetables, whole grains, low-fat milk and plant-based protein rather than meat were 24 percent less likely to have a heart attack and 18 percent less likely to have a stroke than women with more typical U.S. diets. Considering some 40 percent of women over the age of fifty will eventually develop some form of heart disease and stroke, these statistics are very significant.

You will have noted that the diet mentioned above, with its emphasis on fruits, vegetables, whole grains and low-fat milk, pretty well sums up the G.I. Diet. The question of plants—such as soy—rather than meat as the major source of protein is worth noting. Most meats tend to be high in saturated (bad) fats, while protein from plant sources, such as soy, is not. The reality is that most of us are meat eaters, so it is extremely important to ensure you are eating low-fat lean meats such as chicken and fish—in other words, green-light meats—if you are to experience the maximum health benefits.

CANCER

In one of the largest studies to date, British scientists from the University of Manchester pooled information from 221 studies on twenty different cancers. They found conclusive evidence that obesity was replacing smoking as the number-one risk factor for several major cancers. They demonstrated a depressing series of linkages between being overweight and thyroid, kidney, esophageal and colon cancers; multiple myeloma; leukemia; and non-Hodgkin lymphoma in both sexes. It also showed links to rectal cancer and malignant melanoma in men, and gallbladder, pancreas, endometrial and postmenopausal breast cancers in women.

KNEE AND HIP REPLACEMENT

Finally, there is the issue of joint degeneration caused by excessive weight. Just recently the Canadian Institute of Health published a survey of knee and hip replacements performed in Canada in 2004 and 2005. The results showed that not only had the number of operations nearly doubled over the past ten years, but also that overweight and obese patients accounted for a startling 87 percent of knee replacements and 74 percent of hips. Some 54 percent of the knee replacement patients were obese though this group accounts for only 23 percent of the population. Sixty percent of patients were women whose smaller bone structure makes them more vulnerable to extra weight stress. So if you want to reduce your risk of experiencing these leading killer diseases—diabetes, heart disease, stroke, hypertension and cancer—and keep your joints intact—then stay with the program. I can't think of a better motivator.

SLEEP AND WEIGHT LOSS

Overweight people frequently suffer from sleep apnea, which is further complicated for women by menopausal hot flashes. The reason I raise this frustrating issue is that there is increasing evidence that sleep deprivation can cause weight gain; yet another good reason to get a good night's sleep. If hot flashes and/or sleep apnea are seriously interfering with your sleep patterns, then I strongly suggest you see your doctor and ask for advice. While there are many contributors to hot flashes and sleeplessness, it is clear that excessive weight is certainly one that you can do something about.

SUPPLEMENTS

From a dietary standpoint, providing you are eating the green-light way, you are receiving all the nutrients necessary for a healthy life. There are, however, two important exceptions:

VITAMIN D

Vitamin D is known as the sunshine vitamin for very good reason. It is synthesized by the interaction of sunlight on our skin. Its incidence in food is very limited and is primarily confined to fatty fish such as salmon or in fortified milk products.

This vitamin is particularly important for diabetics. Most Type II diabetics have low levels of vitamin D, and a recent Finnish study following 4000 men and women reported people with the highest vitamin D levels had a 40 percent lower risk of developing Type II diabetes as those with the lowest vitamin D levels. Vitamin D deficiency impairs insulin production and resistance.

Vitamin D is also key to reducing your risk for cancer, heart disease and osteoporosis. The problem is that for Canadians sunshine is a scarce commodity in winter, and since we should be lathered in sunscreen during our brief summer we are unable to capitalize on this vitamin self-generation.

Most authorities now recommend a daily supplement of 1000 IU of this inexpensive vitamin.

FISH OIL

There is one oil in particular that has been found to have significant positive health benefits, particularly for your heart. The oil is called omega-3 and it is a fatty acid found primarily in cold-water fish, particularly salmon, as well as a modest amount in canola and flaxseed. As most of us are unlikely to consume salmon on a daily basis, salmon oil is available in capsule form in any pharmacy.

E-CLINIC DIARIES

Many e-clinic members commented about improvements in their health:

> *Depression is an illness that runs deep in my family. I suffer from seasonal affective disorder, and living beside a lake in an isolated area of the Canadian snowbelt doesn't help matters. Every winter, I want to withdraw from the world, comfort myself in ways that are familiar, which includes, of course,*

eating, and eating all the wrong foods to boot . . . I'm trying to fight back, more this year than any other, now . . . that this pre-diabetes diagnosis has been made. I really do find . . . exercise lifts my spirits, which ultimately helps me feel more in control, more determined to change my eating patterns. Not only that, while I'm exercising I'm out of the danger zone (i.e., the kitchen), keeping busy, and not thinking of deprivation. And what's more, exercise suppresses my appetite for quite a while after I finish, and knowing that I'm still burning fat at the same time is empowering . . . and it may be what [I] need to get through a relentlessly long and snowy winter. Bundle up and go for a walk. I highly recommend it. —Kate

I used to get so shaky and anxious from the blood sugar swings and that has really diminished. I find I still get a bit anxious if I haven't eaten in a while but realize now it is not the blood sugar swing but the fear of that swing that is making me anxious. I have started trying to consciously experience hunger and just kind of breathe through the anxiety and let it go. I am setting some new patterns I think will last a lifetime. —Shannon

My husband just had a checkup. His doctor was amazed at how good his blood tests were. He has everything well within the good range for the first time in a long time. (He and I both dropped bad cholesterol 50 to 60 points!) His doc asked him what he was doing to change it, and my husband said, "Just eating what my wife is feeding me!" —Carol

After ten weeks on the plan, I have lost my 10 percent (+ more) that I wanted to lose, 6.5" from my waist, and my blood sugar is down even with dropping most of my meds. I stopped taking glyburide after my first four weeks, and have now gone to two Metformin a day from four. —Ade

The health issues involved with my being overweight and being in a high-risk category to get diabetes are the reasons that I needed to be in this clinic and make myself get serious about trying to prevent some life-threatening diseases. I pray that I didn't start too late. I have always tried to take good care of my health and I always did eat very healthy food, but I also ate things that just tasted wonderful and put on weight. I have also been active and done exercises, but I had a lot of stress in my job. Now that I am retired the stress level has been lowered considerably. What bothers me most is that those of us who are overweight have done this to ourselves and put ourselves in this frightening position!

My goal is to lose the weight, whittle down my waist measurement and get into better shape with more physical activities. I do not want to become a diabetic. I want to do everything in my power to be here for myself and my family for a long time to come. How awful it would be to be dying of some disease and know that I could have done something to possibly prevent it. I want to know that I did my very best and took care of my health. After that, it's up to God.

"You are what you eat" is so true. I know I must eat for my health now and not just for the pleasure in my mouth or the many emotional reasons like I have done in the past.

The statistics for the overweight that put people in the high-risk-health category really scare me and motivate me to drop the old, bad habits and change my way of thinking. I have come a long way during this clinic in the way that I think about and use food. I am very determined to get this weight off for good and then stay on this green-light way of eating for the rest of my life. I have lost the weight before, but I have never been able to keep it off. Now I feel that this is absolutely possible with the G.I. Diet. I have never felt this confident about the future of my weight before. Of course, I still struggle with cravings and the desire to eat like everyone else. But I'm gaining more and more confidence in my future as a thin, healthy person! I can't wait! —Trish

Though exercise is not everyone's favourite topic and has limited value in helping you lose weight, we will show in the next chapter how important it is to your long-term health and weight maintenance.

For Week 11, please see optional meal plan B on pages 177–180 in Part 4.

Week 11 Weight: _____

Week 11 Waist: _____

WEEK 11 DIARY

Week 12
Getting Active

At the beginning of this program, I suggested that weight loss was 90 percent diet and 10 percent exercise, even though exercise is essential for weight maintenance and a healthy lifestyle.

To recap, there are two principal reasons that exercise is not as efficient as diet when you are trying to lose weight. First, it requires a huge amount of effort to burn off those pounds. For example, simply to lose just 1 pound of fat, a 160-pound person would have to walk briskly for 42 miles/67 kilometres or bike 79 miles/127 kilometres! This is something that not many of you are likely to do, even if you physically could.

The following table shows how much exercise effort is required for a 150 pound person to burn off the calories in some popular foods:

Calories and Exercise
One muffin = 2 hours, brisk walking
One granola bar = 1 hour, 10 minutes, jogging
Trail mix (100 g) = 1 hour, 40 minutes, biking
Chocolate bar (half) = 1 hour, 15 minutes, stair machine
One latte = 40 minutes beach volleyball

Food for thought, if you'll pardon the pun!

I'm sure many of you have tried a treadmill or exercise bike at some time and have been amazed at how much effort it takes to burn off even 200 calories. And as you can see, you can blow that and more with just a latte on the way home from the gym.

After much searching I've become aware of the lack of information available in the way of lifestyle help for people who are pre-diabetic or at high risk for heart disease due to weight or body shape. It is most refreshing to have found your book. It's true that I am a very happy customer. I was told I was pre-diabetic a few months ago. With help from a personal trainer and by diligently following your book, my recent blood-work results were an amazing 6.0 (normal).

I understand this will improve if I keep up what I'm doing. I've also lost weight (now 115 pounds) and am changing shape, by reducing belly fat and building muscle. The fact that I actually see results in such a short time is very surprising to me, since I was very skeptical. Thanks to you, we can do something significant to improve our health. —Bonnie

As one pound of fat contains 3,600 calories, you can see why taking the dog for a walk around the block or washing the car has little or no impact on losing weight. Obviously any exercise is better than none, as it all helps to burn extra calories. Just don't expect it to have any significant impact during the weight-loss phase.

The second reason I recommend diet rather than exercise during the weight-loss period is the difficulty obese people—those with a BMI of 30 and over—experience when moving. Quite frankly, I am astonished that many of the big people I have met can actually support their weight. The stress on joints and back carrying an additional 80 to 100 pounds or more is absolutely enormous. Most people couldn't even lift that weight, let alone carry it around all the time. This puts a serious limitation on what overweight people can do to exercise, even if they wanted to.

A recent University of Illinois study clearly demonstrated that exercise decreases insulin resistance. As we are now twelve weeks into the program and many of you have lost sufficient weight, this is the time to consider getting more active. The upside of exercise is that, over the long term, it can help you maintain or accelerate your weight loss, as well as contribute significantly to your health. Diabetics have more to gain from exercise from a health standpoint than most people.

Exercise should become an important consideration particularly for those of you moving from being "obese" to "overweight." Most of you are now better able to exercise as you have less weight to carry around, and you should also be experiencing an increase in your energy levels.

EXERCISE AND MIDDLE AGE

One of the contributors to weight gain as we age is a general reduction in our level of activity. Activities associated with the raising of children are past and the pace of life for most has slowed. However, the accumulation of extra pounds can work against us to reduce the incentive to get off our butts and be active again.

Those of you who decide to do something active are frequently lured by the siren song of fitness clubs that promise a dream body if only you'll sign up. Disappointment is the usual outcome. A principal reason for the very high membership turnover in fitness clubs is their failure to deliver on their promises. Those clubs that empha-size diet as a core component of their program are usually the ones that are more successful.

Now you have your diet under control, have fewer pounds to carry around and more energy, it is time to consider getting more active.

The simplest activity is walking. This doesn't require any special equipment or gym membership, and can be done at virtually any time of the day or year. If you still find it difficult to walk any distance, then a stationary bike is a good investment. The reclining-position bikes are probably easier on your joints as your weight load is spread over a greater area. These are relatively inexpensive and available through many large retail chains such as Walmart or Canadian Tire. Otherwise, join a gym and use the heavy-duty equipment, particularly if your BMI is 30 plus.

My best advice is to incorporate exercise into your daily routine. The easiest way to do this is to follow my "Two Stops Short" program. Simply get off the bus, streetcar or subway two stops short of the office or workplace, and walk. The same in reverse, coming home. If driving, park the car a few blocks away (½ mile/1 kilometre) from the office and walk. Who knows, the parking may be cheaper! This investment of an extra ten minutes a day each way will certainly pay dividends for your weight and health.

I used to do this and found that far from being a drag or inconvenience, I actu-ally looked forward to my "Two Stops Short" walk each day. It helped get me going in the morning and gave me time to reflect on my day with no phones or people crowding me. In the evening, it was a chance to wind down and relax. It required some effort for the first week but quickly became routine for my last three years at the Heart and Stroke Foundation. Try it and let me know how it goes.

In summary then, exercise is of more limited value during the relatively short time period when you are actually losing weight. It is, however, a critical factor in maintaining your weight and health for the rest of your life. Believe it or not, exer-cise can become addictive and I know that I become irritable and edgy if I'm not getting my daily exercise fix—or so Ruth tells me!

Though I have focused on aerobic exercise, the sort of exercise that increases heart rate, there are other important types of exercise. The most important of these are resistance exercises, which are aimed at strengthening your muscles.

MUSCLE MASS

An insidious and silent change that takes place as we age is the loss or thinning of muscle mass. This is a process that starts in our twenties, and by the time women are fifty, and men sixty, they have lost around 15 percent of their muscle mass. From the age of fifty onward the rate of muscle loss escalates quickly. This is due to the decrease in hormone levels and women's increasing inability to convert protein into muscle. Men apparently are able to continue processing protein into muscle, unfair as that might seem.

So why does this loss of muscle mass matter? First, you risk becoming frail as you lack muscle to move and stabilize your body. Without strong muscles in legs and hips, women in particular are at significant risk of debilitating falls and broken bones or worse. In a recent research report on aging and muscle loss, it was stated "if a woman over the age of 65 has a break or fracture from a fall, she has a 50% chance of being dead in two years and that's a frightening statistic."

Second, less muscle means a lower metabolic rate. Muscles are the principal consumer of your body's energy (calories): so the less muscle, the fewer calories you burn and we all know where those surplus calories go. Fat replaces muscle, and fat, conversely, burns fewer calories. However, all is not lost. There are a couple of things you can do to help offset this decline and raise your metabolic rate.

The first is to make sure you are getting adequate protein in your diet. Protein is key to muscle growth and stabilization. The best sources of lean protein are skinless chicken/turkey, fish, eggs (liquid), lean meats, low-fat dairy, soy and legumes (beans). Ideally every snack and certainly every meal should have some protein content. A further benefit of protein is that it slows the digestion and therefore effectively lowers the G.I. of the meal. I often add a scoop of flavoured whey protein powder to my breakfast glass of skim milk, which provides about 25 percent of my daily protein requirement. Orange or strawberry flavours are delicious.

The second offset is exercise. In this instance I do not mean aerobic exercise (i.e., the type of exercise that increases your heart rate such as walking or jogging) but, rather, resistance exercises. In this type of exercise, muscles work against some form of resistance; weights and elastic bands are the two most popular. Resistance exercises are the only ones that build muscle mass. I'm sure most of you associate weights with an image of muscle-bound men sweating and grunting with giant barbells. Don't panic, the reality is far less daunting—even a can of soup can act as a weight.

I don't propose to detail an exact program here, as everyone's needs and budgets are different. Rather, I recommend going to the U.S. Government Center for Disease Control and Prevention site www.CDC.gov/physicalactivity. Click on "Growing stronger—strength training for older adults," and on that page click "Exercises." This is an excellent site that demonstrates how to do various exercises—and it's free!

Boosting your protein intake and adding a few minutes of simple resistance exercises three times a week will go a long way to stabilizing your muscle loss, and, if you are diligent, actually rebuilding some of that loss. You will be less frail and less prone to falling, as well as consuming more calories. Remember, muscles also consume calories when they are at rest and even when you are sleeping.

On a personal note, to give you some encouragement about staying slim and active, my ninety-nine-year-old mother who still lives alone in a two-storey house, has always been active—to the extent that she sometimes trips over her own feet in her haste to get from A to B. This has resulted in two hip fractures as well as two broken arms in the last five years! However, undeterred, she is still mobile and climbs up to her bedroom every evening!

DIABETES AND EXERCISE

Other than getting your doctor's approval to start an exercise program, there are a few other points that are important for diabetics to consider. First, check your blood sugar levels. If they are too low (i.e., 3.3 mmol), or if they are too high (i.e., 13.8 mmol), do not exercise. These figures clearly indicate you are not well, and exercising a sick body is likely to make things worse.

Second, if your blood sugar levels do allow you to exercise, try to do so thirty to sixty minutes after a meal to make sure you have a ready supply of glucose circulating. If you are going to undertake any high-intensity exercise or activities that last for more than thirty minutes, it would be advisable to have a snack on hand to boost your sugar levels.

Finally, if you experience any hypoglycemic symptoms, stop exercising, sit down and check your blood sugar levels. This is where your snack will come in handy. You will quickly learn how much exercise your body can tolerate and adjust accordingly.

Because of the circulatory complications inherent in diabetes, diabetics have more to gain from exercise than most other groups. Regular aerobic exercise (twenty minutes or more, three to five times/week] will improve your blood circulation and therefore reduce your risk of related circulatory diseases such as hypertension, heart disease, stroke, blindness and amputations. I doubt if there is any other single disease that provides as much motivation to get active as diabetes. The ball is in your court.

E-CLINIC DIARIES

Though exercise is not the most efficient way to lose weight, it does increase your metabolic rate and offers a psychological lift. Now is a good time to be considering adding some of the activities discussed here to your routine. It's also a good time to book a retest of your hemoglobin A1C in order to better assess the diet's impact on your blood sugar levels. Here's how our clinic members were feeling at this time:

> *I went to the doctor for my checkup and he was extremely happy with my reports . . . I had lost 12 pounds in four months since I saw him and most of that was with the G.I. life plan. My blood pressure is down. My bone density was above normal in my back and normal in both hips and thighs. The doctor told me to increase my weight-bearing exercises and do balance exercises to keep from falling. He was pleased to hear I was taking vitamin D3 along with calcium for my bones. Although my three-month blood sugar was slightly ele-vated since last time, he was not concerned about it at all since my fasting sugars are regularly low. Thanks!* —Shirley

> *As my body is now accustomed to the time I spend working out, I have gradually increased the time and intensity levels of exercise. While reading* The G.I. Diet *book I recalled how you discovered the VCR again, and I have rediscovered my many CDs, which help me fight off boredom and help time go by as I exercise.* —Sandra

> *I have the problem of pain increasing with exercise due to the fact that I have fibromyalgia and osteoarthritis. I have learned the hard way that I now have to do the exercises less strenuously and build the intensity and duration gradu-ally. I have taken a break from my yoga and walking during this clinic, but I have continued teaching my line-dance class. I have now started to do yoga again, and since I have lost some weight I could definitely feel a difference in my ability to bend more comfortably.*

I prefer to exercise in the privacy of my home. That way I don't have to worry about what to wear or driving to a gym or weather conditions for driving. When the weather is nicer I love to walk outside on the trails. Doing my exercises at home takes much less time because there is no travel time involved. And it costs much less money too! It helps to make exercising fun! Music does it for me as well as variety. I like to set up cross-training activities such as the treadmill, mini trampoline, resistance bands, yoga mat, and floor for dancing and then put the music on and move from one activity to the next.

I also do exercises using DVDs and videos of beginners' yoga and Pilates. I really feel better about myself on the days when I have exercised. Instead of having to think that I should be exercising, I can feel good about the fact that I did exercise that day. —Trish

Exercise . . . is something I have long struggled with. Last winter we purchased a new treadmill and one week into that, I did the splits on the thing. I injured my entire right side and it took months to recover, with the shoulder still not entirely healed.

. . . Now I am back on, with my first goal being a half-hour and that I have met. My next goal is 2 miles an hour and I am at 1.7 going towards 1.8. After that I will work on increasing both time and speed. Want to get to at least 2 ½ miles an hour and [do] an hour several times a week. Also am thinking about starting with free weights but have not done that as yet. One thing that hampered my exercise in the past did that many days I did not feel well enough to be on the treadmill. I finally began to think one of my medications was the culprit, and when I switched to taking it at night, I found that I felt better during the day. —Sharon

I live 3.3 km from work and try to walk at least one way, and both on good days. If I go for a walk at lunch then I am up to 10,000 steps. I have a pedometer, which I find motivating, as I can see my progress. I also try to get to the gym on the weekends and some mornings if I have to take my car to work. It really does make you feel better and is my contemplative time. —Shannon

Well, that's been quite a journey! Some of you will have reached your weight-loss goals or are getting close. Others will be well on their way but are confident they can now stay the course. Either way, next week we will review the top eight lessons from the thirteen-week e-clinic that will help you stay with the program and make it a permanent part of your new lifestyle.

For Week 12, please see optional meal plan B on pages 177–180 in Part 4.

Week 12 Weight: _____

Week 12 Waist: _____

WEEK 12 DIARY

_____

_____

_____

_____

_____

_____

_____

_____

_____

_____

_____

_____

_____

Week 13
Eight Rules for Success

It's useful to review some of the key lessons that we have learnt over the past thirteen weeks, especially as they are the essential building blocks of your future success. I hope you've enjoyed the last thirteen weeks and are feeling healthier, happier and lighter!

> *I started the G.I. Diet after my doctor informed me I had four major problems with my health. My blood pressure, cholesterol, weight over 280 pounds and Type 2 diabetes were dangerous. . . . Well, nine months have passed since I started the G.I. Diet and I now weigh less than 195 pounds and all my health problems are under control or no longer exist. I have lost over 85 pounds and my doctor now calls me his star patient.* —Gail

1. GREEN-LIGHT PANTRY

Clearing red-light foods out of the house and restocking with green-light foods is the single most important step in the program. If those red-light foods aren't there, you won't be tempted. I expect many of you, even after three months, still have those red-light foods around. These are the foods responsible for your weight problem and are poisoning your health. Get them out of your home; they are not your friends.

2. PORTIONS

Portion distortion, or the doubling or even trebling of portion servings over the past twenty years, is one of the principal reasons you have been putting on the pounds. A simple tip is to substitute a lunch-size plate for your dinner plate and remember that the plate should always be $1/2$ vegetables (at least two); $1/4$ protein (meat, fish, chicken or tofu); and $1/4$ rice, potato or pasta. Use moderation and common sense in your portions. Judging from the results to date, you seem to be doing just that.

3. SNACKS

Snacks are critical to the diet as they keep your tummy busy and stop you from getting hungry between meals. Make sure that those snacks are green-light (see Week 2). Always keep in the fridge a plate of sliced vegetables, such as baby carrots, celery, sliced peppers, broccoli florets, along with a tasty hummus dip. This is a staple in our house and our boys now prefer that to their traditional bag of chips.

4. DINING OUT

Whether it's lunch or an evening dining out, you lose some control over what you eat (see Week 8). You are also exposed to greater temptation or choices than at home. However, I've given you the tools to make the right choices, even at McDonald's! Don't be afraid of being assertive. Take control. It's your waistline, your health and your buck. You'll be pleasantly surprised at how cooperative most restaurants will be to reasonable requests. This also may be a chance to show your friends that you are now successfully taking charge of your life.

5. EMOTIONAL EATING

Remember that the original reasons for overeating or using food for comfort may have had origins in our childhood but overeating, negative body image and low self-esteem are the current consequence. And these early psychologically inspired eating behaviours can become eating habits. We eat not only when hungry but also when tired, bored, frustrated, stressed, sad, angry, etc. Stay conscious of your eating habits. Try changing one habit at a time. Work on changing another food-related habit once you feel the first one is under control. Give yourself with a non-food reward for every successful shift in habits (see Week 6).

6. SOCIAL OCCASIONS

This is clearly a difficult challenge for most of you. You don't want to make yourself stand out by eating differently from others and you're concerned that people will see you setting yourself up for failure, again. By now, all of you have shown a commitment and a determination to stay the course to reach your target weight. You are now setting yourself up for success, not failure. Most of you have now lost sufficient weight that the results are beginning to show. No need to hide your success. Share it with your friends. You may be surprised at how supportive they will be when they see the results and realize your determination to succeed.

7. FALLING OFF THE WAGON

This will happen but it's not the end of the world. The G.I. Diet is not a straitjacket and shooting for 90 percent compliance is quite acceptable. Should the fall be a hard one, then you have the tools and knowledge to get back on. Remember the shopping bag motivator/water bottles (Week 5), which I hope you are keeping alongside your scales. It really works. If you haven't done so already, get a friend—or partner—to either join you in losing weight or to be your cheerleader. A friend or partner like this can be a great help in those difficult moments.

> *I am sixty-four years old, and was diagnosed a Type II diabetic six years ago. I've tried every "diet" out there, only to find them unsustainable and unsuccessful in the long run, and was discouraged again and again until I almost gave up even trying! FINALLY I have tried low-glycemic eating, and at last, the weight is coming off, my blood sugar is almost normal, and I feel twenty years younger! A friend told me about your books five years ago—wish I'd listened to her much sooner! The best part is that I am loving this new way of eating. It doesn't feel like dieting at all!* —Sandy

8. EXERCISE

Most of you by now have lost sufficient weight that exercise is starting to become a realistic option (see Week 12). Nearly everyone experiences an increase in their energy levels by this point—because your blood sugar levels have stabilized, and you have fewer pounds to carry around—so you can now get off the couch and start exercising. Walking is the most realistic option for most. Start slowly and gradually increase distance and speed. Although it won't contribute greatly to your weight loss, it will help maintain it, make you feel good and start a healthy habit. Adding some resistance exercises will help you maintain your muscle mass, which starts declining significantly once we reach middle age. Exercise, of course, is essential for your long-term health, especially if you are diabetic.

Since this was the final week of the e-clinic program, most diary entries from this week reflected that. Considering the importance of what the members reported, we decided to devote the next chapter to their results and responses rather than report them here.

For Week 13, please see optional meal plan B on pages 177–180 in Part 4.

Week 13 Weight: _____

Week 13 Waist: _____

WEEK 13 DIARY

_____

_____

_____

_____

_____

_____

_____

_____

_____

_____

_____

_____

_____

_____

_____

_____

_____

Chapter 5
Results of the E-Clinic

Having shared the experiences of the thirty-seven participants for the thirteen weeks of the diabetes clinic, I'm sure you are wondering how they did. First we had a remarkably low dropout rate—less than 10 percent—which is quite impressive given the random selection of participants. Second, for the over 90 percent who completed the thirteen weeks, they all managed to lose weight and inches. Specifically, they lost an average of one pound per week—exactly on target—and an average of three inches from their waist. Most importantly, the average A1C blood sugar measurements fell by nearly 15 percent—and 75 percent of those on medication were able to reduce their dosage. Overall, this is a remarkable achievement after only thirteen weeks.

In this chapter, I will share some of the individual results along with what the participants learned and experienced with the program. As you will see, those who had more weight to lose generally lost weight at a faster rate than those who were closer to their target rate. Space does not allow for either their complete commentaries or for all thirty-seven participants to be included so I've had to make some tough choices, I included these commentaries because I thought they would be most effective at helping you achieve your own goals as they speak to the challenges and successes that participants experienced and that perhaps you will, too!

From Barbara, who lost 15 pounds and 4 inches from her waist, and reduced her A1C from 9.4 to 6.8:

Learning to eat green-light foods is not all that hard. It is now second nature. For the most part I find it easy to stay on program. I am still finding it hard to eat as much as I am supposed to (three snacks a day is a still a little bit much, but I'm finding that part easier as time goes on).

But knowing that you can stray on this program with the 10 percent wiggle room is great. I love chocolate and have found a new favourite (sweet-potato fries). I can give in to my cravings now occasionally (not every day, and not even every weekend) and still feel fine. But, having said that, I find I do not want to have the chocolate and fries like I once did.

But more importantly, I feel a lot better. I do have more energy and have been sleeping better. Before starting the program I had acid reflux every day; now I believe it is a thing of the past. Being perimenopausal, I suffered from hot flashes and night sweats. I cannot say they have disappeared altogether, but they have decreased dramatically. And last week my doctor noticed my weight loss even before I got on the scale.

Exercise was something I put off even after I started this clinic. But now I am walking every evening at least 30 to 45 minutes. It may not sound like much, but that is a great improvement for someone who came home from work, had supper and then just watched TV every night.

Rick, I cannot thank you enough. You have changed my life. I believe I can now look forward to a longer and healthier life.

From Carol, who lost 12 pounds, 3 inches from her waist, and reduced her A1C from 6.9 to 6.4:

Everything is still going in the right direction, down. I like the steady way I lost about a pound a week . . . My husband and I like the diet and don't feel deprived at all. This should be called the low-G.I. lifestyle, not diet! Some authors make G.I. living harder than it really is. They get all hung up on the math of figuring things out. You make it easy . . . for the last three months as my weight went down, so did my blood glucose and especially my bad cholesterol and triglycerides (they have never been this good!). Thank you, Rick, for making the low-G.I. lifestyle easy to follow. People have enough complications in life without having to stumble through a diet of math and counting carbs or points. Your diet is very satisfying and simple to follow. I don't care if it takes a while for me to reach my goals, since I know now how to make this work. I can also accept the fluctuations that life brings, because now I know they are not permanent.

From Cathy, who lost 37 pounds, 7 inches from her waist, and reduced her A1C from 6.3 to 5.6:

I cannot express how amazing this G.I. Diet has been, I have not only lost 37 pounds to date, but I also have been able to manage my blood sugar levels better than I ever had since becoming a diabetic. I have gone from three to four insulin injections a day to two and have been able to go from 24 units per injection to 16. Also I don't need to use a sliding scale of fast-acting insulin . . .

I'm able to enjoy life again without feeling that everything is a struggle and exhausting to do . . . I have made a lifetime change in my diet and will continue to do so . . . If you follow this diet closely your life and health will be truly improved. Believe me because I'm living proof and God knows I feel WONDERFUL and so ALIVE.

From Corinne, who lost 16 pounds, 2 inches from her waist, and reduced her A1C from 7.8 to 6.7:

The G.I. Diet is the simplest, easy to follow way of eating I have every come across. I first read the book Living the G.I. Diet *several years ago. I even tried a few recipes. My sister also had the book and I can remember her and I complaining to each other that "they don't tell you what to eat or how much to eat." I think we were both so used to going on diets that make you count calories, carbs, points or something, that we did not grasp this simple concept. When I was accepted into the e-clinic I ordered and read* The G.I. Diet *book. Suddenly the light bulb went on. I don't comprehend how I had missed the whole point the first time around.*

Support is vital and helps in many ways. I had always made a point of telling no one when I went on diets. That way the failure was my own and didn't have to be shared with anyone. For some reason this time around I decided to tell the world: friends, family, neighbours. I have learned that there is real freedom in having people know what I am doing. If we go out to eat with friends there are no questions of why or how come, although I believe they do watch fairly closely to see what I eat.

I have learned that giving myself permission to make an exception is VERY DANGEROUS and quickly leads me down the slippery slope. I have learned how important it is for me to plan ahead and prepare. When my mom and sisters stayed with me for three days, I had all the main food ready ahead of time, including desserts. All I had to do was make a salad and dinner was ready. Everyone loved the food—I even had some leftovers to send home with Mom. I have learned that it's important for me not to be in a hurry with the numbers. We always say I didn't get this way overnight and can't expect to lose it overnight, but I still felt anxious for the numbers to move faster. I am finally at peace with "slow and easy but surely." I am heading down the right road now and I will get there eventually and safely.

From Gail, who lost 12 pounds, 6 inches from her waist, and reduced her A1C from 6.4 to 6.2:

The most powerful part of this e-clinic for me has been the change in eating habits I have developed. I no longer eat (or want to eat) high-glycemic carbo-hydrates. I have lost my cravings for them. A friend brought over freshly baked chocolate chip cookies this weekend for my family, and while I recognized that they looked good, I had no urge to eat one. Also, last weekend at a friend's house, someone at the dinner table asked me if I wanted a "taste" of cheese-cake. None of me wanted even a taste. It is as though my appetite has shifted. I know I have not been a fast weight loser, but I feel grateful that I have lost steadily and that I am experiencing such a critically important change in crav-ings. Also, I snack or "graze" much less. I plan my snacks, which is entirely different from what I was doing before. I also feel a deepening commitment to my health. These last thirteen weeks have been very stressful (the illness of my mother, some serious health issues for my husband, the moving of my practice to a new office space and Christmas!) and to be able to stay committed to a new way of feeding myself is astonishing to me. With so much OUT of my control, what I can control is my eating and level of exercise. I figure it might take a year or more to be where I'd like, but the time will pass and if I wasn't following the G.I. Diet, I would be heavier and less healthy by year's end.

From Joanne, who lost 22 pounds, 6 inches from her waist, and reduced her A1C from 8.4 to 7.1:

All in all I have to say that I am very pleased that so far this eating plan has worked for me.

What I have learned from this program is to eat smaller portions, eat more frequently, and increase vegetables and fruit in my diet. I have learned that fibre has a big impact on weight loss especially around the waist. My challen-ges at times were trying to fit three meals and two to three snacks into my day. I find that when I am feeling down due to just everyday life struggles and chronic pain, it is hard to think positive and keep on going, but the encourage-ment of your e-mails and the comments of other members are very helpful in keeping me on track.

These last two weeks have been the most challenging and I guess not losing any weight or inches can be considered a failure, but maintaining my weight and not gaining any weight over the last two weeks can be considered somewhat of a success. I refuse to be discouraged by this plateau and will go forward with the hope that the pounds and inches will continue to come off. Thank you, Rick, for this clinic. It has been a lifesaver, as I was spiralling down with my glucose levels and felt helpless to correct the situation mostly because I did not know where to start. I am certain that as I continue on the G.I. Diet, I will achieve my goal of losing weight and getting my glucose levels under control and further reducing my intake of medication, hopefully even getting off of medication, and being healthy.

From Kate, who lost 14 pounds, 3 inches from her waist, and reduced her A1C from 8.0 to 7.2:

Many times in the past I would say to myself that I didn't care that I was overweight, that I accepted myself as I was, that my health was not affected to any great degree. (I had high blood pressure, but there are no outward symptoms, right?) But with my pre-diabetes diagnosis, I knew that my health was seriously compromised and could become more precarious if I didn't take any steps to stop the relentless deterioration. I was finding I couldn't chase the ball with my kids anymore, hated putting my bathing suit on, was starting to sit on the sidelines as the rest of my family skied, hiked, skated. Did I want to look back on my life as a bystander, an observer? The window of opportunity for sharing experiences with my kids in their childhood was starting to close. How could I squander this chance for living to the fullest? And if I didn't arrest the path of diabetes and obesity, I could develop more serious diseases and cut my life expectancy by untold years. Getting control over the power food has over you is what it's all about, bottom line. And that may be one of the hardest things you do because it may be a lifelong struggle. Fattening food has held sway over me for most of my life. Eating sweets is one of my favourite things to do, no doubt about it. But the question I have had to ask was: Is it worth my health; is it worth denying myself life's other pleasures? Undoubtedly, the answer is NO.

All the rules of the G.I. Diet make perfect sense. In my experience, it is the most sensible, safe and healthful approach to weight loss and it is a way of eating and thinking that could be sustained reasonably for a lifetime. And the thing is, I do believe you don't have to deny yourself the pleasures of eating.

But you do have to educate yourself, and your palate, and your pleasure sensors and that takes the will to change. Like all endeavours worth doing, the journey is fraught with challenges and hardships, but in the end it's worth it. I want that kind of success for myself and my family. Now I feel more energetic, I feel encouraged and I feel more in control of my life. So, what have I learned along the way? It's all about choices and about digging deep to make the right ones.

From Pat, who lost 14 pounds, 2 inches from her waist, and reduced her A1C from 6.4 to 6.2:

The G.I. Diet has been the most successful diet for me. It is based on safe, sensible and easy-to-understand (at least for me) scientific research that doesn't lose sight of other aspects of a person's health by seeking only weight loss. There are no special foods or wacky combinations or deprivation tactics involved—just healthy food that is readily available and suits every budget. Three meals, three snacks a day, balanced and healthy choices—what could be simpler! Many weight-loss programs just didn't work for me because as long as I can remember, I have had to eat at regular times through the day or I would suffer the consequences of sugar highs and lows. Without knowing about the glycemic index and the way sugar affects my body I was destined to continue on the wrong track. Although I have been watching fats, cholesterol, eating fruit and vegetables, and cut way back on salt and sugar anyway, it still didn't have the effect that the G.I. Diet has had.

The changes I have had to make in my diet have been relatively small, but monumentally successful. It has now become second nature to choose foods that work for me. I will have to struggle a bit when my daughter is home from school over the summer, but I feel that the next couple of months will give me a chance to solidify my way of eating so that I don't let myself be sabotaged. Permanently losing weight in a healthy way is full of roadblocks, challenges and pitfalls along the way. Emotional eating is a huge one for me and until I addressed it, I would have stayed in the same old patterns. I can sincerely say if I can do this and stick with it, anybody can.

I love the feeling I get when I see and feel the effects of this clinic. Carrying that grocery bag of weight equivalent to what I have lost is one of the best exercises I have ever done and I continue to do it regularly—it is a great way to measure success in an instant. I am lighter, happier, healthier, wearing smaller clothing, receiving compliments about my weight loss and can actually feel my ribs and hip bones again!!! The scientific and personal support I have gotten from this experience will enable me to live a healthier and, hopefully, longer life. For that, I can't thank you enough.

From Sandra, who lost 29 pounds, 7 inches from her waist, and reduced her A1C from 8.0 to 4.0:

"The word credo is Latin for "I believe." Here is my G.I. Credo:

I believe in three balanced meals and two snacks per day.

I believe in low-glycemic foods.

I believe that foods with high glucose increase my blood sugar level.

I believe that I have the ability to be the best I can be.

I believe that I am the only one who controls what I put in my mouth and what eventually grows on my belly.

I realize that I should chew my food carefully and put down my fork between bites.

I realize that caffeine is a stimulant and increases adrenaline levels and increases appetite.

I realize that excessive weight puts undue stress on my joints and back.

I realize that I have 10 percent wiggle room on the G.I. Diet.

In order to be successful one has to be organized and cook and prepare staples beforehand.

A plate should be 50 percent vegetables, 25 percent good carbs and 25 percent protein.

Exercise can be and should be fun. Once your body adjusts to the routine, the intensity and duration should be increased.

From Trish, who lost 12 pounds, 1 ½ inches from her waist, and reduced her A1C from 5.9 to 4.7:

There have been many things that I've learned or improved during the last 12 weeks in this clinic.

1. The song "Love the One You're With" comes to mind because I've learned to enjoy the green-light foods that I can eat and not worry about the red-light foods that I shouldn't have because they are not healthy for me anyway.

2. I love that I can find a delightful green-light substitute for almost any food I may want, but shouldn't have, so I don't have to mourn the loss of any food.

3. Support from others is very helpful but making this way of eating successful has to come from within ME. I also know that I have to constantly nurture and refresh this drive within to stay motivated. Remember, what you eat in private shows in public!

4. A big benefit of this diet is that I don't have to weigh and measure and record everything that I eat each day. This is a huge time saver. But, I've also learned that since I don't have to do that, I have to be very careful about the following point.

5. Portion Control! This is an area that needs constant regulation on my part. It's too easy to have just a bit more because the food is green-light and delicious. There are so many wonderful recipes and choices in the G.I. plan, that I have to be very vigilant and not eat too much. For me, this is a daily test.

6. I've learned that I have to eat the green-light way the rest of my life. I am pre-diabetic with insulin resistance and I have to do everything in my power to never cross over to being a diabetic. I have to work hard and do my part. After that, it's up to God.

7. One of my biggest successes is the change in my cravings. The comfort foods I used to crave are no longer comfortable! They were making me ill and overweight and I don't crave them so much anymore. I know this will be a life-long struggle, but it gets better all the time. Just the thought of eating some, or too much, of the formerly craved foods makes me remember how badly I would feel if I did that now. I enjoy the feeling of better health that I experience now. I try to think of sugar as something that poisons my body.

8. I've learned that I have to be my own food monitor and check in my G.I. books regularly to review daily menus, green-light choices and limited portion sizes for some foods. I have to be vigilant with this because this is my health. I can never become complacent about any of this knowledge.

9. I also have to be aware of eating patterns from the past that led to my being overweight and continue to find ways to change each bad habit into a healthy habit. This self-awareness is a soul-searching journey and will also be ongoing. I know it's all too easy to slip back into old patterns. Each time I conquer any past slip-ups I give myself a pat on the back for a job well done!

10. I've learned that I have to keep my motivation high especially when the weight is very slow to go down. When I feel as if I'm going nowhere, I check my weight-loss graph and see the progress as it shows a stairway in a steady descent over the past few months. This visual of the progress I've made gives me the stamina I need to keep on this journey. It shows me that persistence pays off in the long run.

11. I have really enjoyed being in this clinic for many reasons. It helped me to finally get serious about losing weight and becoming healthier. As I said at the very beginning, it was the kick in the butt that I needed. It has helped me begin to change many bad eating habits that were holding me back even though I also ate very healthy food.

PART III: Week 14 and Beyond

Chapter Six
Where to Go from Here

Whether you have reached your weight-loss target by now and are ready to start Phase II of the G.I. Diet, or still have some way to go, you may find some helpful ongoing support on my clinic website, www.gidietclinic.com, which includes a series of nine monthly newsletters as well as an online forum to share your experiences with other readers.

The e-clinic is a great opportunity to continue your past experience with the G.I. Diet. Whether you join the e-clinic or not, I would be delighted to hear about your experiences. Simply e-mail me at Rick@gidiet.com.

PHASE II

Well, you've made it. Congratulations! You've hit your target weight, you're digging out clothes you thought you'd never get into again, and you're finally on good terms with your full-length mirror. I hope you are relishing the new you and making the most of your increased energy. Now that you've graduated from Phase I, you can ease up a bit on limiting portion and serving sizes, and start adding some yellow-light foods to your diet. The idea here is to get comfortable with your G.I. program; this is how you're going to eat for the rest of your life.

The best news for most of us in Phase II is about alcohol and chocolate. While both were considered red-light in the Preliminary Phase and Phase I because of their high calorie content and tendency to spike blood sugar levels, in Phase II, it's time to reintroduce those little pleasures.

ALCOHOL

Medical research indicates that red wine, which is rich in flavonoids, can help reduce your risk of heart disease and stroke. So, in Phase II, a glass of red wine is allowed with dinner. Just because one glass is beneficial, however, doesn't mean that two or three is even better for you. Immoderate drinking undoes any health benefits, and alcohol contains calories. One glass of wine (5 ounces maximum) provides the optimum benefit.

Apart from red wine, keep your consumption of alcohol to a minimum. I realize that this can be difficult, since drinking is so often a part of social occasions and celebrations. An occasional lapse won't do a lot of harm, but it's easy to get carried away. There are various strategies to combat the social pressure to drink: you can graciously accept that glass of wine or cocktail, raise it in a toast, take a sip, and then discreetly leave it on the nearest buffet table. Faced with a tray of vodka martinis and glasses of red wine, stick with the wine, which lasts longer. Ruth drinks spritzers (wine mixed with soda water) on special occasions. And if you add lots of ice to your spritzer, you can reduce the alcohol even further while still joining in the party spirit. Whatever strategy you choose, always try to eat some food with your drink, even if it has to be a forbidden piece of cheese. The fat will slow the absorption of the alcohol and minimize its impact. (Of course, better to gravitate to the vegetable tray, but an emergency canapé won't be the ruin of you.)

CHOCOLATE

For many of us, living without chocolate is not living. The good news is that in Phase II, some chocolate—the right sort of chocolate in the right amount—is acceptable. You may have heard that chocolate, like red wine, contains natural elements that help keep the arteries clear—but that's probably not your main motive for eating it! Chocolate combines fat, sugar and cocoa, all three of which please the palate. But most chocolate contains too much saturated fat and sugar, which keeps it deep in the red-light zone. Chocolate with a high cocoa content (70 percent or more) delivers more chocolate intensity per ounce, which means that even a square or two is satisfying. A square or two can give chocoholics the fix we need.

TO SUM UP

- In Phase II, use moderation and common sense in adjusting portions and servings.
- Don't view Phase II as a straitjacket. Occasional lapses are fine.

GREEN-LIGHT SERVINGS

PHASE II

Chocolate (at least 70 percent cocoa)	2 squares
Red wine	One 5-ounce glass

MODERATION IS KEY

Phase II, I must warn you, is a bit of a danger zone, the stage when most diets go off the rails. Most people think that when they reach their weight-loss goal, they can just drop the diet and go back to their old eating habits. And frankly, when I take a close look at what many of these diets expect you to live on, I can understand why people can't stick to them for long.

The reality is that, with some modifications, the G.I. Diet program is your diet for life. But this shouldn't be a hardship, because the G.I. Diet was designed to give you a huge range of healthy choices, so you won't feel hungry, bored or unsatisfied. By now, you will know how to navigate your green-light way through the supermarket, decipher food labels and cook the green-light way. You are probably not even tempted to revert to your old ways. If you should fall prey to a double cheeseburger, you will be dismayed at how heavy, sluggish and ungratified you feel afterward. You will be too attached to your new feeling of lightness and level of energy to abandon them.

Before we look at some of the new options open to you in Phase II, a word of caution: your body can now function on less food than it did before you started. Why? Because you're lighter now, so your body requires fewer calories. Also, your metabolism has become more efficient, and your body has learned to do more with fewer calories. Keeping these two developments in mind, add a few more calories in Phase II, but don't go berserk. Don't make any significant changes in your serving sizes, and remember to make yellow-light foods the exception rather than the rule. This way, you will keep the balance between the calories you're consuming and the calories you're expending—and that is the secret to maintaining your new weight.

As you modestly increase portions of foods that you particularly enjoy and include some yellow-light items as a treat, keep monitoring your weight weekly, and adjust your servings up or down until your weight stays stable. This may take a few weeks of experimentation, but when you've reached the magic balance and can stay there comfortably, that's the formula for the rest of your days.

Here are some ideas of how you might alter the way you eat in Phase II.

BREAKFAST
- Increase cereal serving size from 1/2 to 2/3 of a cup.
- Add a slice of 100% whole-grain toast and a pat of margarine.
- Double the amount of sliced almonds on your cereal.
- Enjoy an extra slice of back bacon.
- Have a glass of unsweetened juice now and then.
- Add one of the yellow-light fruits—a banana or apricot—to your cereal.
- Go caffeinated in the coffee department, if you like, but try to keep it to one cup a day.

LUNCH
I suggest you continue to eat lunch as you did in Phase I, as this is the one meal that already contained some compromises in the weight-loss portion of the program.

DINNER
- Add another boiled new or small potato.
- Increase the pasta serving from 3/4 cup to 1 cup.
- As a special treat, have a 6-ounce steak instead of a 4-ounce one.
- Eat a few more olives and nuts—but only a few!
- Try a cob of sweet corn with a dab of margarine.
- Add a slice of high-fibre bread or crispbread.
- Enjoy a yellow-light cut of lamb or pork.

SNACKS
- Have a maximum of 2 cups of microwavable, light popcorn.
- Increase your serving size of nuts to 10 or 12.
- Enjoy a square or two of 70 percent dark chocolate.
- Have a banana.
- Indulge in a scoop of low-fat ice cream or frozen yogurt.

Of course, Phase II is not, and shouldn't be, a straitjacket. If you live 90 percent within the guidelines of the diet, you are doing well. The idea that certain foods are completely and forever forbidden would drive you, sooner or later, back into their clutches. With the G.I. Diet, you are in control of what you eat, and that includes (with discipline, moderation and common sense) almost everything.

PART IV: Meal Plans and the Recipes

MEAL PLANS

Following you will find four basic meal plans, each with an accompanying grocery list that provides all you need to make the week's worth of food. These meal plans are both optional and flexible, and repeat over weeks 5 through 14—a note at the end of each week tells you to which meal plan you should refer. While some people who prefer a fully structured program might follow each day to the letter, others might prefer to plan their own green-light meals and snacks, using the meal plan only as a guide. You'll soon get to know which are your favourites!

OPTIONAL MEAL PLAN A

Note: You are not required to use these weekly meal plans and shopping lists.

Feel free to pick and choose and make up your own green-light meals.

	BREAKFAST	SNACK	LUNCH	SNACK	DINNER	SNACK
MON	Hot Oatmeal with Pears and Dried Cranberries (p. 191)	Cranberry Cinnamon Bran Muffin (p. 257)	Open-faced Chicken Sandwich with lettuce, tomato and onion, and Basic G.I. Salad (p. 211)	Laughing Cow Light cheese with crispbread	Lemon Linguine with Smoked Salmon (p. 235), Broccoli and Salad	Mixed berries tossed in lime juice with sour cream
TUES	Mini Breakfast Puffs (p. 195)	Fruit Yogurt	G.I. Pasta Salad (p. 215)	Hummus with carrot and celery sticks	Cheesy Lentil and Bean Bake (p. 223), basmati rice and salad	Orange and almonds
WED	G.I. Granola (p. 192)	Slice of Banana Bread (p. 258) and glass of skim milk	Broccoli, Sun-Dried Tomato and Feta Quiche (p. 226)	Baby Gouda Lite cheese with crispbread	White Chicken Chili (p. 241), rice and salad	Cran-Apple Oatmeal Bar (p. 268) and glass of skim milk

THURS	Hot Oatmeal (p. 191)	Small apple and glass of skim milk	Quick and Easy Chicken Noodle Soup (p. 203) and Basic G.I. Salad (p. 211)	Crunchy Chickpeas (p. 256)	Miso-Crusted Salmon (p. 234) with asparagus	½ Nutrition bar
FRI	All-Bran Buds with skim milk, peace slices and sliced almonds	Fruit yogurt	Mixed Bean Salad (p. 217)	Laughing Cow Light cheese with crispbread	Beef Cutlets in Mushroom Gravy (p. 251), new potatoes, green beans and salad	Mixed berries tossed in lime juice with sour cream
SAT	Smoked Salmon Scrambled Eggs (p. 199)	½ Nutrition bar	Cottage cheese Salad (p. 213)	Hummus with carrot and celery sticks	Orange Chicken with almonds (p. 243), green beans and basmati rice	Creamy Raspberry Mousse (p. 263)
SUN	Oatmeal Buttermilk Pancakes with strawberries (p. 194)	Orange and almonds	Caesar Salad (p. 212) with canned tuna	Babybel Gouda Lite cheese with crispbread	Vegetarian Moussaka (p. 230) with basmati rice	Piece of Rhubarb-Ginger Cobbler (p. 265)

GROCERY LIST FOR MEAL PLAN A

PRODUCE
Almonds (whole and sliced)
Apple rings (dried)
Apples
Asparagus
Bananas
Broccoli
Cabbage
Carrots
Celery
Cranberries (dried)
Cucumbers (English and field)
Eggplant
Fresh herbs (chives, cilantro, dill, flat-leaf
    parsley, oregano, thyme)
Garlic
Ginger root
Green onions
Jalapeño
Kale
Lemons
Lettuce (iceberg, leaf and romaine)
Limes
Mushrooms
Onions (yellow and red)
Oranges
Peaches (fresh or canned in juice or water)
Pears (Bosc or Bartlett)
Peppers (green, red or yellow)
Potatoes (new or small)
Radishes
Raisins
Raspberries

Rhubarb (fresh or frozen)
Strawberries
Sunflower seeds (shelled and unsalted)
Tomatoes (plum)

DELI
Hummus
Lean deli chicken
Olives (black or green)
Sun-dried tomatoes

BAKERY
100% stone ground whole wheat bread
Crispbread (e.g., Wasa Fiber)
Whole-grain bread
Whole wheat bread crumbs
Whole wheat crackers
Whole wheat pita bread

FISH COUNTER
Salmon fillets
Smoked salmon

MEAT COUNTER
Chicken breast (boneless, skinless)
Chicken sausage (lean)
Ground beef (extra lean)
Ground turkey (lean)

**BEANS (LEGUMES) AND
CANNED VEGETABLES**
Black beans
Cannellini (white kidney) beans

Chickpeas
Diced tomatoes
Lentils (green)
Mixed beans
Tomato paste

PASTA AND SAUCES
Light tomato sauce (no added sugar)
Linguine (whole wheat)
Rotini or penne (whole wheat)
Small pasta (e.g., ditali or tubetti)

SOUP AND CANNED SEAFOOD AND MEAT
Anchovy fillets
Beef broth (low-fat, low-sodium)
Chicken stock (low-fat, low-sodium)

GRAINS AND SIDE DISHES
Basmati rice
Flaxseed (ground)

INTERNATIONAL FOODS
Mirin (or sweet sherry)
Sesame seeds
Soy sauce (low-sodium)
Tahini
White miso

COOKING OIL, VINEGAR, SALAD DRESSINGS AND PICKLES
Dijon mustard
Oil (canola, extra-virgin olive and sesame)
Red wine vinegar
Rice vinegar

Salsa
Worcestershire sauce

SNACKS
Applesauce (unsweetened)
Nutrition bars (e.g., ZonePerfect, Balance Bar)

BAKING
Baking powder
Baking soda
Cornstarch
Honey
Spices (allspice, cayenne, Cajun seasoning, ground cinnamon, ground cumin, curry powder, ground nutmeg, dried oregano, black pepper, red pepper flakes, salt, dried thyme)
Splenda
Vanilla
Wheat bran
Whole wheat flour

BREAKFAST FOODS
All-Bran Buds or 100% Bran cereal
Oatmeal (large-flake oats)
Steel-cut oats

BEVERAGES
Amaretto
White wine

DAIRY CASE
Babybel Gouda Lite cheese
Buttermilk

Cheddar cheese (low-fat)

Cottage cheese (1%)

Egg whites

Feta cheese (light)

Fruit yogurt (non-fat with sweetener)

Laughing Cow Light cheese (extra-low-fat)

Liquid eggs (e.g., Naturegg Break Free)

Milk (skim)

Soft margarine (non-hydrogenated, light)

Sour cream (low-fat)

Whole Omega-3 eggs

Yogurt (low-fat)

FROZEN FOODS

Orange juice concentrate

Peas (or fresh)

Raspberries

OPTIONAL MEAL PLAN B

	BREAKFAST	SNACK	LUNCH	SNACK	DINNER	SNACK
MON	Hot Oatmeal with Pears and Dried Cranberries (p. 191)	Slice of Banana Bread (p. 258) and glass of skim milk	Open-faced lean deli ham sandwich with lettuce, tomato, red pepper and grainy mustard, and Basic G.I. Salad (p. 211)	Laughing Cow Light cheese with crispbread	Citrus-Poached Haddock (p. 233) with asparagus, carrots and new potatoes	Mixed berries tossed in lime juice with sour cream
TUES	Bacon and Egg Muffin (p. 196)	Fruit Yogurt	Winter Vegetable Soup with Spinach (p. 205) and Basic G.I. Salad (p. 211)	Hummus with carrot and celery sticks	Bolognese Pasta sauce (p. 253) with whole wheat pasta and Basic G.I. Salad (p. 211)	Orange and almonds
WED	G.I. Granola (p. 192) with skim milk and fruit yogurt	Cranberry Cinnamon Bran muffin (p. 257)	Cottage cheese with apple and grapes, and Basic G.I. Salad (p. 211)	Baby Gouda Lite cheese with crispbread	Chicken Tarragon with mushrooms (p. 244), broccoli and basmati rice	Chocolate Pudding (p. 267) and glass of skim milk

THURS	Hot Oatmeal with Pears and Dried Cranberries (p. 191)	Small apple and glass of skim milk	Tuna Salad (p. 216)	Crunchy Chickpeas (p. 256)	Cheesy Lentil and Bean Bake (p. 223)	½ Nutrition bar
FRI	All-Bran Buds with skim milk, peach slices and sliced almonds	Fruit yogurt	½ Whole wheat pita with deli turkey, lettuce, tomato and cucumber, and Basic G.I. Salad (p. 211)	Laughing Cow Light cheese with crispbread	Ginger-Wasabi Halibut (p. 237), Cold Noodle Salad with Cucumber and Sesame (p. 214), snow peas and carrots	Creamy Raspberry Mousse (p. 263)
SAT	Breakfast in a glass (p. 197)	½ Nutrition bar	Crab Salad in Tomato Shells (p. 219)	Hummus with carrot and celery sticks	Chicken Tikka (p. 239), snow peas, rice or bulgur and salad	Chocolate Pudding (p. 267) and glass of skim milk
SUN	Cinnamon French Toast (p. 193) with back bacon	Orange and almonds	Minestrone (p. 201) and Basic G.I. Salad (p. 211)	Babybel Gouda Lite cheese with crispbread	Grilled Portobello Mushroom Pizzas (p. 225) and salad	Slice of Apple Raspberry Coffee Cake (p. 266)

GROCERY LIST FOR MEAL PLAN B

PRODUCE
Almonds
Apples
Asparagus
Bananas
Carrots
Celeriac
Celery

Cranberries (dried)
Cucumbers (English and field)
Fresh herbs (basil, chives, cilantro, dill,
   flat-leaf parsley, oregano, tarragon)
Garlic
Ginger root
Grapes
Kale

Lemons

Lettuce (iceberg, leaf and romaine)

Limes

Mushrooms (Portobello and plain)

Onions (yellow and red)

Oranges

Peaches (fresh or canned in juice or water)

Pears (Bosc or Bartlett)

Pecans

Peppers (green, red or yellow)

Potatoes (new or small)

Raspberries

Snow peas

Spinach (baby)

Strawberries

Sweet potato

Tomatoes (large beefsteak and plum)

DELI

Hummus

Lean deli ham

Lean deli turkey

Olives (black or green)

BAKERY

100% stone ground whole wheat bread

Crispbread (e.g., Wasa Fibre)

Whole-grain bread

Whole wheat pita bread

FISH COUNTER

Frozen crab

Haddock fillets

Halibut fillets

MEAT COUNTER

Back bacon

Chicken breast (boneless, skinless)

Ground beef (extra lean)

BEANS (LEGUMES) AND CANNED VEGETABLES

Black beans

Chickpeas

Crushed tomatoes

Diced tomatoes

Lentils (green)

Plum tomatoes

PASTA AND SAUCES

Ditali or tubetti (whole wheat)

Fettuccine or Linguine (whole wheat)

SOUP AND CANNED SEAFOOD AND MEAT

Chicken stock (low-fat, low-sodium)

Tuna (light, in water)

Vegetable stock (low-fat, low-sodium)

GRAINS AND SIDE DISHES

Basmati rice

Bulgur

Flaxseed (whole and ground)

Sunflower seeds

INTERNATIONAL FOODS

Mirin (or sweet sherry)

Rice vinegar

Sesame seeds

Soy sauce (low-sodium)

Wasabi powder

COOKING OIL, VINEGAR, SALAD DRESSINGS AND PICKLES

Capers

Dijon mustard

Dry mustard

Grainy mustard

Mayonnaise (fat-free)

Oil (canola and extra-virgin olive)

Red wine vinegar

SNACKS

Nutrition bars (e.g., ZonePerfect, Balance Bar)

BAKING

Baking powder

Baking soda

Brown Splenda

Cocoa powder

Cornstarch

Honey

Soy lecithin granules

Spices (chili powder, garam masala, ground cumin, ground cinnamon, ground nutmeg, dried oregano, black pepper, red pepper flakes, dried rosemary, salt, dried thyme, turmeric)

Splenda

Vanilla

Wheat bran

Wheat or soy protein isolate powder

Whole wheat flour

BREAKFAST FOODS

All-Bran Buds and 100% Bran cereal

Steel-cut oats

BEVERAGES

Amaretto

Red wine

Vermouth or white wine

DAIRY CASE

Babybel Gouda Lite cheese

Buttermilk

Cheddar cheese (low-fat)

Cottage cheese (1%)

Fruit yogurt (non-fat with sweetener)

Laughing Cow Light cheese (extra-low-fat)

Liquid eggs (e.g., Naturegg, Break Free)

Milk (skim)

Soft margarine (non-hydrogenated, light)

Sour cream (low-fat)

Soy milk

Whole Omega-3 eggs

Yogurt (low-fat)

FROZEN FOODS

Mixed berries

Orange juice concentrate

Raspberries

OPTIONAL MEAL PLAN C

	BREAKFAST	SNACK	LUNCH	SNACK	DINNER	SNACK
MON	Hot Oatmeal with Pears and Dried Cranberries (p. 191)	Apple Bran Muffin (p. 259)	Open-faced sandwich with lettuce, tomato and onion, and Basic G.I. Salad (p. 211)	Laughing Cow Light cheese with crispbread	Lemony Grilled Vegetable Pasta (p. 209) with canned tuna or salmon	Mixed berries tossed in lime juice with sour cream
TUES	Mini Breakfast Puffs (p. 195)	Fruit yogurt	Tuscan White Bean Soup (p. 202) with Basic G.I. Salad (p. 211)	Hummus with carrot and celery sticks	Spicy Roasted Chicken with Tomatoes and Tarragon (p. 245), green beans and basmati rice	Orange and almonds
WED	G.I. Granola (p. 192) with skim milk and fruit yogurt	Apple Bran Muffin (p. 259)	½ Whole wheat pita with canned light tuna, lettuce, tomato and cucumber, and Basic G.I. Salad (p. 211)	Baby Gouda Lite cheese with crispbread	Pork Medallions Dijon (p. 254), green beans, carrots and new potatoes	Creamy Lemon Square (p. 270) and glass of skim milk
THURS	Hot Oatmeal with Pears and Dried Cranberries (p. 191)	Small apple and glass of skim milk	Quick and Easy Chicken Noodle Soup (p. 203) and Basic G.I. Salad (p. 211)	Crunchy Chickpeas (p. 256)	Grilled TLT Sandwich (p. 224) and Basic G.I. Salad (p. 211)	½ Nutrition bar
FRI	All-Bran Buds with skim milk, peach slices and sliced almonds	Fruit yogurt	Waldorf Chicken and Rice Salad (p. 218)	Laughing Cow Light cheese with crispbread	Thai Red Curry Shrimp Pasta (p. 236)	Mixed berries tossed in lime juice with sour cream

SAT	Vegetarian Omelette (p. 198)	½ Nutrition bar	Cottage Cheese Salad (p. 213)	Hummus with carrot and celery sticks	Zesty Barbecued Chicken (p. 246) and Tangy Red and Green Coleslaw (p. 210)	Creamy Lemon Square (p. 273) and glass of skim milk
SUN	Oatmeal Buttermilk Pancakes (p. 194) with strawberries	Orange and almonds	Tuna Salad (p. 216)	Babybel Gouda Lite cheese with crispbread	G.I. Fish Fillet (p. 237) with broccoli and cauliflower tossed in lemon juice	Piece of Rhubarb-Ginger Cobbler (p. 265)

GROCERY LIST FOR MEAL PLAN C

PRODUCE

Almonds

Apples

Broccoli

Cabbage (green and red)

Carrots

Cauliflower

Celery

Cranberries (dried)

Cucumbers (English and field)

Eggplant

Fresh herbs (basil, chives, dill, cilantro, marjoram, oregano, flat-leaf parsley, rosemary, sage, tarragon, thyme)

Garlic

Ginger root

Green beans

Green onions

Kale

Lemons

Lettuce (iceberg, leaf and romaine)

Limes

Mushrooms (shiitake)

Onions (yellow and red)

Oranges

Pears (Bosc or Bartlett)

Peppers (green, red or yellow)

Potatoes (new or small)

Radishes

Rhubarb (fresh or frozen)

Raisins

Shallots

Strawberries

Tomatoes (cherry and plum)

Walnuts

Zucchini

DELI
Hummus (light)
Kalamata olives

BAKERY
100% stone ground whole wheat bread
Crispbread (e.g., Wasa Fiber)
Whole-grain bread
Whole wheat pitas
Whole wheat tortillas

FISH COUNTER
Fish fillets
Shrimp (large, raw)
Smoked salmon

MEAT COUNTER
Chicken breast (boneless, skinless)
Pork tenderloin

BEANS (LEGUMES) AND CANNED VEGETABLES
Chickpeas
Extra-firm tofu
Kidney beans (red and white)
Tomato paste

PASTA AND SAUCES
Penne or rotini (whole wheat)
Small pasta (e.g., ditali or tubetti)
Spaghettini or linguine (whole wheat)
Light tomato sauce

SOUP AND CANNED SEAFOOD AND MEAT
Chicken stock (low-fat, low-sodium)

Tuna (light, in water)
Vegetable stock (low-fat, low-sodium)

GRAINS AND SIDE DISHES
Basmati rice
Flaxseed (ground)

INTERNATIONAL FOODS
Rice vinegar
Sesame seeds
Soy sauce (low-sodium)
Thai red curry paste

COOKING OIL, VINEGAR, SALAD DRESSINGS AND PICKLES
Buttermilk salad dressing (low-fat, low-sugar)
Capers
Cider vinegar
Dijon mustard
Oil (canola, extra- virgin olive and sesame)
Red wine vinegar
Worcestershire sauce

SNACKS
Applesauce (unsweetened)
Nutrition bars (e.g., ZonePerfect, Balance Bar)

BAKING
Baking powder
Baking soda
Cornstarch
Honey
Oat bran
Spices (ground allspice, celery seeds,

chili powder, ground cinnamon,
ground cloves, ground nutmeg, black
pepper, salt)
Splenda
Vanilla
Wheat bran
Whole wheat flour

BREAKFAST FOODS
All-Bran Buds cereal
Steel-cut oats

BEVERAGES
Vermouth or white wine

DAIRY CASE
Buttermilk
Cheddar cheese (light)

Cottage cheese (1%)
Egg whites
Extra-firm tofu
Feta cheese (light)
Laughing Cow Light cheese (extra-low-fat)
Liquid eggs (e.g., Naturegg, Break Free)
Milk (skim)
Soft margarine (non-hydrogenated, light)
Sour cream (low-fat)
Whole Omega-3 eggs
Yogurt (low-fat)

FROZEN FOODS
Apple juice concentrate
Mixed berries
Orange juice concentrate
Peas (or fresh)

OPTIONAL MEAL PLAN D

	BREAKFAST	SNACK	LUNCH	SNACK	DINNER	SNACK
MON	Hot Oatmeal with Pears and Dried Cranberries (p. 191)	Whole Wheat Fruit Scone (p. 260)	Open-faced lean deli ham sandwich with lettuce, tomato, red pepper and grainy mustard, and Basic G.I. Salad (p. 211)	Laughing Cow Light cheese with crispbread	Fettuccine Primavera (p. 229) and Caesar Salad (p. 212)	Mixed berries tossed in lime juice with sour cream
TUES	Bacon and Egg Muffin (p. 196)	Fruit yogurt	Waldorf Chicken and Rice Salad (p. 218)	Slice of Banana Bread (p. 258) and glass of skim milk	Stuffed Peppers (p. 249) and Basic G.I. Salad (p. 211)	Orange and almonds

WED	G.I. Granola (p. 192) with skim milk and fruit yogurt	Whole Wheat Fruit Scone (p. 260)	Broccoli, Sun-dried Tomato and Feta Quiche (p. 226), and Basic G.I. Salad (p. 211)	Babybel Gouda Lite cheese with crispbread	Chicken Schnitzel (p. 242), green beans, carrots and new potatoes	Cran-Apple Oatmeal Bar (p. 268) and glass of skim milk
THURS	Hot Oatmeal with Pears and Dried Cranberries (p. 191)	Small apple and glass of skim milk	Minestrone Soup (p. 201) and Basic G.I. Salad (p. 211)	Crunchy Chickpeas (p. 256)	Meatloaf (p. 250), green beans, carrots and new potatoes	½ Nutrition bar
FRI	All-Bran Buds with skim milk, peach slices and sliced almonds	Fruit yogurt	½ Whole wheat pita with deli turkey, lettuce, tomato and cucumber, and Basic G. I. Salad (p. 211)	Laughing Cow Light cheese with crispbread	Indian Vegetable Curry (p. 228) and Basic G.I. Salad (p. 211)	Fancy Fruit Salad (p. 263)
SAT	Smoked Salmon Scrambled Eggs (p. 199)	½ Nutrition bar	Cottage Cheese with apple and grapes, high-fibre crackers and Basic G.I. Salad (p. 211)	Hummus with carrot and celery sticks	G.I. Fish Fillet (p. 237) and Lemony Stir-Fried Vegetables (p. 222), new potatoes, asparagus and Basic G.I. Salad (p. 211)	Creamy Raspberry Mousse (p. 263) and glass of skim milk
SUN	Cinnamon French Toast (p. 193) with back bacon	Orange and almonds	Grilled Shrimp and Pear Salad (p. 220)	Babybel Gouda Lite cheese with crispbread	Chicken Stir-Fry and Broccoli (p. 240) and Basic G.I. Salad (p. 211)	Chocolate Pudding (p. 267) with berries

GROCERY LIST FOR MEAL PLAN D

PRODUCE

Almonds

Apricots

Apples

Asparagus

Bananas

Bean sprouts

Blackberries

Blueberries (fresh or frozen)

Broccoli

Carrots

Cashews

Celery

Cranberries (dried)

Cucumbers

Fresh herbs (basil, chives, cilantro, dill,
    oregano, flat-leaf parsley, mint, thyme)

Garlic

Ginger root

Grapes

Green beans

Green onions

Kiwis

Lemons

Lettuce (iceberg, leaf and romaine)

Limes

Mushrooms (shiitake)

Onions (yellow, red and vidalia)

Oranges

Peaches (fresh or canned in juice or water)

Pears (Bosc or Bartlett)

Peppers (green, red or yellow)

Potatoes (new or small)

Snow peas

Spinach (baby)

Strawberries

Sunflower seeds (shelled and unsalted)

Tomatoes (large beefsteak and plum)

Walnuts

Zucchini (yellow and green)

DELI

Hummus (light)

Lean deli ham

Lean deli turkey

Parmesan cheese, grated

Sun-dried tomatoes

BAKERY

100% stone ground whole wheat bread

Crispbread (e.g., Wasa Fiber)

High-fibre crackers

Whole-grain bread

Whole wheat bread crumbs

Whole wheat pita bread

FISH COUNTER

Fish fillets

Frozen crab

Smoked salmon

MEAT COUNTER

Back bacon

Chicken breast (boneless, skinless)

Ground beef (extra-lean)

BEANS (LEGUMES) AND CANNED VEGETABLES

Chickpeas

Kidney beans (red)

Lentils

Plum tomatoes

Tomato paste

PASTA AND SAUCES

Small pasta (e.g., ditali or tubetti)

Fettuccine or linguine (whole wheat)

SOUP AND CANNED SEAFOOD AND MEAT

Anchovy fillets

Chicken stock (low-fat, low-sodium)

Vegetable stock (low-fat, low-sodium)

GRAINS AND SIDE DISHES

Barley

Basmati rice

INTERNATIONAL FOODS

Hoisin sauce

Oyster sauce

Rice vinegar

Sesame seeds

Soy sauce (low-sodium)

Tahini

COOKING OIL, VINEGAR, SALAD DRESSINGS AND PICKLES

Buttermilk salad dressing (low-fat, low-sugar)

Dijon mustard

Grainy mustard

Oil (canola, extra-virgin olive and sesame)

Worcestershire sauce

SNACKS

Applesauce (unsweetened)

Nutrition bars (e.g., ZonePerfect, Balance Bar)

BAKING

Baking powder

Baking soda

Cocoa powder

Cornstarch

Oat bran

Spices (ground cinnamon, cumin seeds, curry powder, ground cloves, ground nutmeg, dried oregano, black pepper, red pepper flakes, salt)

Splenda

Vanilla

Wheat bran

Wheat germ

Whole wheat flour

BREAKFAST FOODS

All-Bran Buds cereal

Steel-cut oats

BEVERAGES

Amaretto

Tomato juice

Vegetable cocktail juice

DAIRY CASE

Babybel Gouda Lite cheese

Buttermilk

Cheddar cheese (low-fat)

Cottage cheese (1%)

Egg whites

Feta cheese (light)

Fruit yogurt (non-fat with sweetener)

Laughing Cow Light cheese (extra-low-fat)

Liquid eggs (e.g., Naturegg, Break Free)

Milk (skim)

Soft margarine (non-hydrogenated, light)

Sour cream (low-fat)

Tofu (firm)

Whole Omega-3 eggs

FROZEN FOODS

Mixed berries

Orange juice concentrate

Raspberries

THE RECIPES

BREAKFAST

Hot Oatmeal with Pears and Dried Cranberries

A satisfying hot breakfast for when there's a chill in the air. You can substitute apples, peaches or nectarines for the pears, and instead of dried cranberries, try using other dried fruits or a mixture of a few different kinds. Oats can be toasted and stored in an airtight container at room temperature up to 1 week. Refrigerate finished oatmeal up to 1 day. Reheat, adding a little more milk or water to thin to desired consistency.

1 cup	steel-cut oats
2 cups	skim milk
2 cups	water
2 pears	(Bosc or Bartlett), cored and chopped
½ cup	dried cranberries
1 tsp	cinnamon
¼ tsp	nutmeg
	Splenda (optional)

1. Preheat oven to 300°F.

2. Place oats on rimmed baking sheet and toast in oven for 20 minutes. In large saucepan, combine milk and water and bring to boil. Stir in oats, pears, cranberries, cinnamon and nutmeg and return to boil. Reduce heat to low and cook, stirring occasionally, for 20 minutes or until thickened and oats are tender. Stir in Splenda to taste, if desired.

Makes 4 servings.

G.I. Granola

There are so many uses for this granola beyond serving it for breakfast with skim milk or low-fat yogurt: sprinkle it on fruit salad or low-fat, no-sugar ice cream, or eat a couple of handfuls as a snack. You can store in an airtight container at room temperature up to 2 days or freeze up to 1 month.

2 cups	large-flake oats
1 cup	dried apple rings, chopped (or ½ cup dried cranberries or raisins)
½ cup	sunflower seeds
½ cup	sesame seeds
½ cup	almonds, chopped
½ cup	ground flaxseed
1 tbsp	cinnamon
2 tsp	grated orange zest
½ tsp	salt
1	egg white
1 tbsp	canola oil
1 tbsp	honey
2 tsp	frozen orange juice concentrate
1 tsp	vanilla

1. Preheat oven to 350°F.

2. In large bowl, mix together oats, apple, sunflower seeds, sesame seeds, almonds, flax-seed, cinnamon, orange zest and salt.

3. In small bowl, whisk together egg white, oil, honey, orange juice concentrate and vanilla. Pour into oat mixture and toss until thoroughly coated. Turn out onto parchment paper–lined rimmed baking sheet and spread evenly. Bake, turning mixture once with spatula halfway through, for 25 to 30 minutes or until mixture is golden brown.

Makes about 6 cups (12 servings).

Cinnamon French Toast

Serve this family favourite with slices of ham or back bacon and extra strawberries for a complete breakfast.

³⁄₄ cup	liquid egg
¹⁄₂ cup	skim milk
1 tbsp	Splenda
1 tsp	vanilla
¹⁄₂ tsp	ground cinnamon
Pinch	salt
4 slices	stone-ground whole wheat bread
1 tsp	canola oil
2 cups	sliced strawberries
¹⁄₂ cup	non-fat sugar-free fruit-flavoured yogurt

1. In shallow dish, whisk together liquid egg, milk, Splenda, vanilla, cinnamon and salt. Dip each slice of bread into egg mixture, making sure to coat both sides.

2. Meanwhile, brush oil onto non-stick griddle or large non-stick frying pan over medium-high heat. Cook for about 4 minutes, turning once, or until golden brown. Serve with strawberries and yogurt.

Makes 2 servings.

Oatmeal Buttermilk Pancakes

Make pancake breakfasts a weekend tradition. Serve them with fresh fruit or applesauce.

³⁄₄ cup	large-flake oats
2 cups	buttermilk
1 cup	whole wheat flour
¹⁄₄ cup	ground flaxseed
1 tbsp	Splenda
1 tsp	ground cinnamon
1 tsp	baking soda
1 tsp	baking powder
¹⁄₄ tsp	salt
¹⁄₂ cup	liquid egg
2 tbsp	canola oil
1 tsp	vanilla

1. In bowl, soak oats in buttermilk for 20 minutes.

2. In large bowl, combine flour, flaxseed, Splenda, cinnamon, baking soda, baking powder and salt.

3. In another bowl, whisk together liquid egg, oil and vanilla. Stir in soaked oats and buttermilk. Pour over flour mixture and stir until just mixed.

4. Meanwhile, heat non-stick griddle or large non-stick frying pan over medium heat. Ladle about ¹⁄₄ cup batter onto griddle for each pancake. Cook until bubbles appear on top, about 2 minutes.

5. Flip pancakes and cook for another 2 minutes or until golden. Transfer to plate and cover to keep warm. Repeat with remaining batter.

Makes 16 pancakes, 4 to 6 servings.

Mini Breakfast Puffs

Ideal for rushed mornings, these muffin-sized puffs are packed with nutrition.

1 tsp	canola oil
¼ cup	diced onion
1	red pepper, diced
1 cup	chopped broccoli
1 ½ tsp	fresh thyme
¼ tsp	each salt and freshly ground pepper
¾ cup	crumbled light feta cheese
1 ½ cups	liquid egg
1 cup	skim milk
¼ cup	wheat bran
¼ cup	whole wheat flour

1. Preheat oven to 400°F.

2. In non-stick frying pan, heat oil over medium heat. Cook onion and red pepper for about 5 minutes or until softened. Add broccoli, thyme, salt and pepper; cover and steam for about 3 minutes or until broccoli is tender-crisp and bright green. Divide mixture among 12 greased muffin tins.

3. Sprinkle cheese over top of vegetable mixture in each cup.

4. In bowl, whisk together liquid egg, milk, bran and whole wheat flour. Divide evenly over vegetable mixture. Bake for about 20 minutes or until golden, set and puffed. Let cool slightly before serving.

Makes 12 puffs, 6 to 8 servings.

Bacon and Egg Muffin

Two of these muffins make a delicious portable breakfast. You can wrap muffins individually in plastic wrap and refrigerate up to 2 days or freeze up to 1 month. Reheat in microwave for 30 seconds on high.

1 tsp	olive oil
1	onion, chopped
1	small jalapeño pepper, finely chopped (optional)
4 slices	peameal bacon or ham, chopped
1 can (420 mL)	artichoke hearts, drained and chopped
¾ cup	wheat bran
½ cup	shredded light-style Swiss cheese
¼ cup	chopped fresh basil or parsley
1 ½ cups	liquid egg
¾ cup	skim milk
1 tsp	freshly ground pepper

1. Preheat oven to 350°F. Line 12 muffin tins with paper or foil liners.

2. In non-stick frying pan, heat oil over medium-high heat. Cook onion and jalapeño, if using, for 5 minutes or until softened. Transfer to bowl and allow to cool for 5 minutes. Stir in bacon, artichokes, wheat bran, cheese and basil.

3. In separate bowl, whisk together egg, milk and pepper. Pour into bacon and onion mixture and stir until well combined.

4. Carefully ladle into muffin tins, filling to top.

5. Bake for 25 minutes or until filling is firm and tops are slightly brown. Let cool on rack for 5 minutes. Carefully remove muffins from tin and allow to cool completely.

Makes 12 muffins.

Breakfast in a Glass

This is a great make-and-take breakfast for mornings on the run. It packs protein, fruit and fibre in one glass. Look for whey or soy protein isolate in your local health food store.

¼ cup	flaxseed
2 tbsp	sunflower seeds
2 cups	soy milk
2 cups	fresh or frozen berries
½	banana
½ cup	low- fat yogurt
½ cup	whey or soy protein isolate powder
2 tbsp	soy lecithin granules (optional)

1. In spice or coffee grinder, finely grind flaxseed and sunflower seeds. Set aside.

2. In blender or food processor, blend together soy milk, berries, banana and yogurt until almost smooth.

3. Add seed mixture, protein powder and lecithin, if using, to soy milk mixture. Blend just until mixed, about 5 seconds.

Makes 2 servings.

Vegetarian Omelette

A good basic recipe. you can change the taste by switching up the seasoning. Instead of pepper, try oregano and basil or red pepper.

1 tsp	canola oil
1 cup	broccoli florets
½ cup	sliced mushrooms
½ cup	chopped red and green pepper
½ cup	liquid egg
1 oz	low-fat cheddar cheese, shredded
Pinch	freshly ground pepper

1. In small non-stick frying pan, heat oil over medium-high heat. Add broccoli, mushrooms and pepper, and sauté until tender, about 5 minutes. Transfer vegetables to a plate and cover to keep warm.

2. In bowl, using fork, stir together liquid egg, cheese and pepper. Pour into frying pan and cook for about 5 minutes, lifting edges to allow uncooked egg to run underneath, until almost set.

3. Sprinkle sautéed vegetables over half of the omelette. Using spatula, fold over other half and cook for 1 minute.

Makes 1 serving.

Smoked Salmon Scrambled Eggs

Smoked salmon makes scrambled eggs elegant and special. Serve with a slice of high-fibre toast.

4	egg whites
2	omega-3 eggs
2 tbsp	skim milk
¼ tsp	freshly ground pepper
1 tsp	canola oil
2 oz	smoked salmon, chopped
1 tbsp	chopped fresh chives or dill

1. In bowl, whisk together egg whites, eggs, milk and pepper.
2. In non-stick frying pan, heat oil over medium heat. Add egg mixture. Using rubber spatula, gently stir eggs until almost set. Stir in salmon and continue to cook, stirring gently, until eggs are set but still slightly creamy. Stir in chives.

Makes 2 servings.

SOUPS

Minestrone Soup

This soup is one of my favourites because it contains both pasta and spinach. Serve it with a sprinkling of grated Parmesan cheese for extra flavour and a few more red pepper flakes to get your blood pumping.

2 tsp	canola oil
3 slices	back bacon, chopped
1	onion, chopped
4 cloves	garlic, minced
2	carrots, chopped
1 stalk	celery, chopped
1 tbsp	dried oregano
½ tsp	red pepper flakes
¼ tsp each	salt and freshly ground pepper
1 can (796 mL)	plum tomatoes
6 cups	chicken stock (low-fat, low-sodium)
1 bag (300 g)	baby spinach washed well
1 can (540 mL) each	red kidney beans and chickpeas, drained and rinsed
¾ cup	ditali or tubetti pasta
⅓ cup	chopped fresh flat-leaf parsley (optional)
2 tbsp	chopped fresh basil (optional)

1. In large soup pot, heat oil over medium-high heat and cook back bacon for 2 minutes. Reduce heat to medium and add onion, garlic, carrots, celery, oregano, red pepper flakes, salt and pepper. Cook for about 10 minutes or until vegetables are softened and lightly browned.

2. Add tomatoes and crush using potato masher in pot. Pour in chicken stock; bring to boil. Reduce heat to simmer and add spinach, beans, chickpeas and pasta. Simmer for 6 to 10 minutes or until pasta is tender. Stir in parsley and basil (if using).

Makes 6 servings.

Tuscan White Bean Soup

Serve this soup in deep Italian ceramic soup bowls and dream you're in Tuscany.

1 tbsp	extra-virgin olive oil
1	onion, chopped
4 cloves	garlic, minced
1	carrot, chopped
1 stalk	celery, chopped
4	fresh sage leaves or ½ tsp dried
6 cups	vegetable or chicken stock (low-fat, low-sodium)
2 cans	cannellini or white kidney beans, drained and rinsed
(540 mL each)	
4 cups	shredded kale
Pinch each	salt and freshly ground pepper

1. In large soup pot, heat oil over medium heat. Add onion, garlic, carrot, celery and sage and cook for 5 minutes or until softened.

2. Add stock, beans, kale, salt and pepper, and cook, stirring occasionally, for about 20 minutes or until kale is tender.

Makes 6 to 8 servings.

Quick and Easy Chicken Noodle Soup

Why buy canned soup when you can make this simple homemade version?

2 tsp	extra-virgin olive oil
2	carrots, chopped
2 stalks	celery, chopped
3 cloves	garlic, chopped
1	onion, chopped
1 tbsp	chopped fresh thyme
6 cups	chicken stock (low-fat, low-sodium)
3	boneless skinless chicken breasts (4 oz each), diced
1 cup	frozen peas
¾ cup	small pasta (such as ditali or tubetti)
¼ cup	chopped fresh flat-leaf parsley
¼ tsp each	salt and freshly ground pepper

1. In large soup pot, heat oil over medium-high heat. Add carrots, celery, garlic, onion and thyme, and cook for 10 minutes or until vegetables are slightly softened.

2. Pour in stock and bring to boil. Reduce heat to simmer and add chicken. Cook for 5 minutes, then add pasta and peas. Cook until pasta is al dente and chicken is no longer pink. Stir in parsley, salt, pepper.

Makes 6 servings.

Ham and Lentil Soup

Canned lentils make this soup quick and easy to prepare, so keep some on hand. If you want to make this soup even more green-light, use dried lentils (see instructions at the bottom of this page).

1 tbsp	canola oil
1	onion, chopped
1 cup	diced celery
2	cloves garlic, minced
6 cups	chicken stock (low-fat, low-sodium)
2 cans (540 mL each)	lentils, drained and rinsed
6 oz	black forest ham, diced
1	red pepper, diced
2	tomatoes, seeded and diced
2 tbsp	chopped flat-leaf parsley

1. In large soup pot, heat oil over medium heat. Add onion, celery and garlic, and cook for about 5 minutes or until softened. Add stock, lentils, ham and red pepper; bring to boil. Reduce heat and add tomatoes. Cover and simmer for 20 minutes. Stir in parsley.

Makes 6 servings.

Variation: Use 1 cup dried green or brown lentils. Add with stock, and cover and simmer for about 30 minutes or until tender.

Winter Vegetable Soup with Spinach

A nutritious soup to fend off winter's chill.

2 tsp	olive oil
3	medium carrots, chopped
2 cloves	garlic, chopped
1	onion, chopped
1 lb	celeriac (also known as celery root), chopped
1	large sweet potato, chopped
1 tsp	dried thyme
½ tsp	dried rosemary
6 cups	chicken or vegetable stock (low-fat, low-sodium)
¾ cup	small pasta (such as ditali or tubetti)
½ tsp each	salt and freshly ground pepper
1 bag (10 oz)	baby spinach

1. In large soup pot, heat oil over medium-high heat. Cook carrots, garlic, onion, celeriac, sweet potato, thyme and rosemary for 8 minutes or until vegetables are starting to soften and turn golden.

2. Pour in stock and bring to boil. Reduce heat, cover and simmer, stirring occasionally, for 25 minutes or until vegetables are tender.

3. Working in batches, purée soup in blender or food processor until smooth, then return to pot. Bring to boil and add pasta, salt and pepper. Reduce to a simmer and cook for about 5 minutes. Add spinach and cook for another 5 minutes or until pasta is tender.

Makes 6 servings.

G.I. Pesto

The addition of water along with the oil in this pesto reduces the fat content. It gives the pesto a lighter green colour than traditional pesto, but it still tastes great.

2 cups	packed fresh basil leaves
3 cloves	garlic
1/3 cup	sunflower seeds
1/4 cup	grated Parmesan cheese
1 1/2 tbsp	lemon juice
1/4 tsp each	salt and freshly ground pepper
3 tbsp	water
3 tbsp	extra-virgin olive oil

1. In blender or food processor, purée basil, garlic, sunflower seeds, Parmesan, lemon juice, salt and pepper. With motor running, add water and oil in steady stream.

Makes 3/4 cup.

Make Ahead: Refrigerate in airtight container up to 3 days or freeze up to 6 months.

Helpful Hint: When basil is plentiful, make extra batches and freeze in ice-cube trays. When frozen, remove from tray and store in airtight container in freezer. You'll always have a bit of pesto on hand to stir into hot pasta or soups.

SALADS

Raita Salad

This recipe is based on the refreshing Indian condiment. Try serving this salad with Chicken Tikka (see recipe, page 239).

1 bag (300 g)	baby spinach washed well
1	medium English cucumber, quartered lengthwise and sliced into ½-inch chunks
2	tomatoes, chopped
½	red onion, thinly sliced
1 cup	low-fat plain yogurt
½ tsp	ground cumin
¼ tsp	salt

1. In large bowl, toss together spinach, cucumber, tomatoes and red onion.
2. In another bowl, stir together yogurt, cumin and salt. Add to spinach mixture and toss to coat.

Makes 4 servings.

Lemony Grilled Vegetable Pasta Salad

This is a lovely side dish for chicken or fish. Toss in some leftover roast chicken or a can of tuna or salmon for a simple lunch. The salad can be refrigerated for up to 3 days.

⅓ cup	chopped shallots
¼ cup	olive oil
¼ cup	lemon juice
2 tbsp	Dijon mustard
2 tbsp	chopped fresh herbs (choose from a mixture of thyme, rosemary, oregano and marjoram)
1 tbsp	grated lemon zest
¼ tsp each	salt and freshly ground pepper
1	small eggplant, quartered, then cut crosswise into ½-inch-thick slices
1 each	red pepper and yellow pepper, seeded and cut into ½-inch pieces
1	zucchini, halved and cut into ½-inch rounds
1	red onion, cut into wedges
1	carrot, cut into ¼-inch-thick rounds
6 oz	shiitake mushrooms (discard stems, cut caps in four)
3 cups	whole wheat penne or other similar-size pasta shape
2 tbsp	chopped fresh basil or parsley

1. Preheat oven to 425°F.

2. In large bowl, whisk together shallots, oil, lemon juice, mustard, herbs, lemon zest, salt and pepper. Add eggplant, peppers, zucchini, onion, carrot and mushrooms and toss with dressing. Place on rimmed baking sheet and roast in oven for 25 to 30 minutes or until vegetables are golden and tender.

3. Meanwhile, in large pot of boiling salted water, cook pasta for 8 minutes or until al dente. Drain and add cooked vegetables and basil, tossing well.

Makes 4 to 6 servings.

Tangy Red and Green Coleslaw

Using a vinaigrette in coleslaw makes it low-fat and really tangy! This is a great keeper salad for the refrigerator or to tote along to a potluck.

4 cups	finely shredded green cabbage
2 cups	finely shredded red cabbage
2	carrots, shredded
½ cup	thinly sliced celery
¼ cup	chopped fresh flat-leaf parsley
½ cup	cider vinegar
2 tbsp	canola oil
2 tsp	Splenda
1 tsp	celery seeds
½ tsp	salt
Pinch	freshly ground pepper

1. In large bowl, toss together green and red cabbage, carrots, celery and parsley.
2. In small bowl, whisk together vinegar, oil, Splenda, celery seeds, salt and pepper. Pour over cabbage mixture and toss to coat.

Makes 4 to 6 servings.

Basic G.I. Salad

Both the salad and the dressing in this recipe can be prepared ahead and stored separately, covered, for about 2 days.

1 ½ cups	lettuce (try any type) torn or coarsely chopped
1	small carrot, grated
½	red, yellow or green pepper, diced
1	plum tomato, cut into wedges
½ cup	sliced cucumber
¼ cup	chopped red onion (optional)

Basic G.I. Vinaigrette:

1 tbsp	vinegar (try any type) or lemon juice
1 tsp	extra-virgin olive oil or canola oil
½ tsp	Dijon mustard
1 clove	garlic, crushed (optional)
Pinch each	salt and freshly ground pepper
Pinch	finely chopped fresh herb of choice

1. In large bowl, toss together lettuce, carrot, pepper, tomato, cucumber and onion.
2. In small bowl, whisk together vinegar, oil, mustard, garlic, salt, pepper and herb.
3. Pour vinaigrette over greens and toss to coat.

Makes 1 serving.

Variation: To make a meal out of salad, add protein with 4 oz canned tuna, cooked salmon, tofu, kidney beans, chickpeas, cooked chicken or another lean meat.

Caesar Salad

We all need a Caesar salad in our recipe repertoire. No one will guess that tahini is the secret ingredient that makes this green-light version every bit as creamy as Chef Caesar Cardini's original.

3 slices	whole-grain bread
2 tsp	extra-virgin olive oil
Pinch each	salt and freshly ground pepper
1	large head romaine lettuce

Dressing:

3 cloves	garlic, minced
3	anchovy fillets, finely minced
2 tbsp	tahini
1 tsp	Dijon mustard
½ tsp	Worcestershire sauce
½ tsp each	salt and freshly ground pepper
3 tbsp	fresh lemon juice
2 tbsp	warm water
1 ½ tbsp	extra-virgin olive oil

1. Preheat oven to 350°F.
2. Cut bread into ½-inch pieces and place in bowl. Add oil, salt and pepper and toss to coat well. Arrange in single layer on rimmed baking sheet. Bake for 20 minutes or until golden and crisp. Let cool.
3. Wash lettuce and tear into bite-sized pieces; place in large bowl.
4. In small bowl, stir together garlic, anchovies, tahini, mustard, Worcestershire sauce, salt and pepper. Whisk in lemon juice, water and oil.
5. Pour dressing over lettuce and toss to coat. Sprinkle with croutons.

Makes 4 servings.

Cottage Cheese Salad

This creamy, crunchy salad can also be stuffed into a whole wheat pita.

2 cups	low-fat cottage cheese
½ cup	grated carrot
½ cup	grated celery
½ cup	grated radish
2	green onions, chopped
1	large apple, cored and chopped
2 tsp	minced fresh ginger
2 tsp	soy sauce
1 clove	garlic, minced
1 tsp	rice vinegar
½ tsp	toasted sesame oil

1. In bowl, stir together cottage cheese, carrot, celery, radish, green onions, apple, ginger, soy sauce, garlic, vinegar and sesame oil.

Makes 4 servings.

Cold Noodle Salad with Cucumber and Sesame

These refreshing noodles pair well with Ginger-Wasabi Halibut (see recipe, page 237).

6 oz	thin pasta (vermicelli, capellini or spaghettini)
1 tbsp	rice vinegar
4 tsp	Splenda
2 tsp	soy sauce (low-sodium)
½	English cucumber, quartered lengthwise and thinly sliced
2 tbsp	toasted sesame seeds

1. In large pot of boiling salted water, cook pasta until al dente, about 4 minutes. Drain and rinse under cold water. Place in large bowl.

2. In small bowl, stir together vinegar, Splenda and soy sauce. Pour over cooked noodles, and stir in cucumber and sesame seeds; toss well to coat.

Makes 6 servings.

G.I. Pasta Salad

No summer buffet for a crowd is complete without a pasta salad. Use seasonal vegetables as they become available. Vary the vegetables, sauce and source of protein to suit you tastes and add variety to your pasta salads.

½ to ¾ cup	cooked whole wheat pasta (spirals, shells or similar size)
1 cup	chopped cooked vegetables (such as broccoli, asparagus, peppers or green onions)
¼ cup	light tomato sauce or other low-fat or non-fat pasta sauce
4 oz	cooked chicken or other lean meat, such as lean ground turkey or lean chicken sausage, chopped

1. Place the pasta, vegetables, tomato sauce and chicken in a bowl and stir to mix well. Refrigerate, covered, until ready to use, then heat in the microwave or serve chilled.

Makes 1 serving.

Tuna Salad

This mixture is also nice served in endive spears or romaine lettuce leaves.

1 can (19 oz)	cannellini (white kidney) beans, drained and rinsed
1 clove	garlic, minced
2 cans (6 oz each)	chunk light tuna, drained
1	large tomato, chopped
¼ cup	capers
2 tbsp	chopped fresh parsley
1 tbsp	lemon juice
¼ tsp each	salt and freshly ground pepper
4 slices	whole-grain bread

1. Using potato masher, in bowl mash half of the cannellini beans with garlic. Coarsely chop remainder of beans.

2. In another bowl, mix tuna, beans, tomato, capers, parsley and lemon juice. Stir in bean mixture and salt and pepper.

3. Divide mixture evenly among bread slices.

Makes 4 servings.

Mixed Bean Salad

This salad can be a meal all on its own or with some protein like tuna or cooked chicken.

1 can (540 mL)	mixed beans, drained and rinsed
½	cucumber, chopped
1	tomato, chopped
1 cup	cooked whole wheat pasta (small shells, macaroni or similar size)
2 tbsp	chopped fresh flat-leaf parsley
1 tbsp	red wine vinegar
2 tsp	extra-virgin olive oil
¼ tsp	Dijon mustard
Pinch each	salt and freshly ground pepper
Pinch	finely chopped fresh herbs (such as thyme or oregano)

1. Place beans in large bowl and add cucumber, tomato, pasta and parsley.
2. In small bowl, whisk together vinegar, oil, mustard, salt, pepper and herbs. Pour over salad and toss to coat.

Makes 2 servings.

Waldorf Chicken and Rice Salad

A green-light twist on a classic salad, this makes a delicious lunch.

³/₄ cup	cooked basmati or brown rice
1	medium apple, chopped
1 or 2	celery stalks, chopped
¹/₄ cup	walnuts
4 oz	cooked chicken, chopped
1 tbsp	store-bought light buttermilk dressing

1. Place rice, apple, celery, walnuts and chicken in large bowl. Pour in buttermilk dressing and stir to mix.

Makes 1 serving.

Crab Salad In Tomato Shells

Beefsteak tomatoes are ideal for this dish because their large size will accommodate the filling, and pulp and seeds are easy to scoop out.

2 packages (200 g each)	frozen crab, thawed
4	large beefsteak tomatoes
¼ cup	fat-free mayonnaise
2 tbsp	low-fat sour cream
½ tsp	grated lemon zest
1 tbsp	fresh lemon juice
2 tsp	chopped fresh tarragon
Pinch each	salt and freshly ground pepper
1 cup	coarsely chopped cooked chickpeas
½	red pepper, diced
¼ cup	finely diced celery
¼ cup	chopped fresh flat-leaf parsley
2 tbsp	chopped fresh chives
2 tbsp	shredded carrot

1. Place crab in fine-mesh sieve; press out any liquid. Remove and discard any cartilage if necessary; set aside crab.

2. Cut top quarter off tomatoes. Using small spoon, scoop out seeds and pulp, and discard. Place tomatoes cut side down on paper towel–lined plate.

3. In large bowl, stir together mayonnaise, sour cream, lemon zest and juice, tarragon, salt and pepper. Add chickpeas, red pepper, celery, parsley, chives and carrot. Add crab and stir to combine. Divide crab mixture among tomatoes.

Makes 4 servings.

Grilled Shrimp and Pear Salad

This light dish from our friend Meryle combines unexpected ingredients to yield delicious results.

4	pears, quartered, cored and sliced
1	red pepper, seeded and chopped
1	red onion, chopped
¼ cup	chopped cilantro
1 lb	large raw shrimp, peeled and deveined
1 tbsp	canola oil
1 tsp	chopped fresh oregano

Dressing:

2 tbsp	rice vinegar
2 tbsp	orange juice
1 tsp	orange zest
1 tsp	honey or maple syrup

1. Preheat oiled grill or broiler to high.
2. In large bowl, whisk together vinegar, orange juice, orange zest and honey.
3. Add pears, red pepper, red onion and cilantro to dressing; toss to coat. Set aside.
4. In bowl, toss shrimp with oil and oregano. If you plan to grill the shrimp, thread onto bamboo skewers that have been soaked in water for 30 minutes. If you plan to broil them, spread on baking sheet. Grill or broil shrimp, turning once, until pink and firm, about 4 minutes.
5. Divide salad mixture among plates and top with shrimp.

Makes 4 to 6 servings.

MEATLESS

Lemony Stir-Fried Vegetables

The lemon really enhances the flavour of this easy vegetable dish.

2 tsp	canola oil
10	shiitake mushrooms, stemmed and sliced
2	carrots, thinly sliced on the diagonal
1	red, yellow, green or orange pepper, sliced
1	zucchini, halved lengthwise and sliced on the diagonal
1 tbsp	minced fresh ginger
1 clove	garlic, minced
2 cups	snow peas, trimmed
4	green onions, sliced on the diagonal
	zest and juice of 1 lemon
1 tbsp	soy sauce
¼ cup	toasted sesame seeds

1. In wok or large non-stick frying pan, heat oil over medium-high heat. Add mushrooms, carrots, red pepper, zucchini, ginger and garlic. Stir-fry for 2 to 3 minutes.

2. Add snow peas and green onions. Stir-fry for another 2 to 3 minutes or until vegetables are tender-crisp.

3. Stir in lemon zest and juice and soy sauce. Cook for 1 minute. Sprinkle in sesame seeds, tossing to coat vegetables.

Makes 4 to 6 servings.

Cheesy Lentil and Bean Bake

If you'd like, you can stir in the meat shredded from one smoked turkey drumstick (look in the deli section of the supermarket) before putting the lentil and bean mixture in the baking dish. Serve with basmati rice or pasta.

1 cup	dried green lentils (preferably du Puy), rinsed
1 tbsp	olive oil
1	onion, chopped
4 cloves	garlic, chopped
1 can (796 mL)	diced tomatoes
4 cups	chopped kale (tough stems removed)
2 tsp	Cajun seasoning*
½ tsp	salt
1 can (540 mL)	black beans (or pinto beans), drained and rinsed
1 cup	shredded light-style cheddar cheese

1. Preheat oven to 375°F.

2. In saucepan, cook lentils in 3 cups water for 20 to 30 minutes or until soft. Drain and set aside.

3. Meanwhile, in large non-stick frying pan, heat oil over medium-high heat; cook onion and garlic until softened, about 5 minutes. Add diced tomatoes, kale, Cajun seasoning and salt; cook, stirring occasionally, for 10 minutes or just until kale is tender. Stir in lentils and beans.

4. Spread mixture in 13- × 9-inch glass baking dish and sprinkle cheese evenly over top. Bake for 20 minutes or until cheese is melted and mixture is bubbling.

Makes 6 servings.

* If Cajun seasoning is unavailable, make your own by combining 2 tsp each cumin, chili powder, dried basil, dried oregano, dried mustard, paprika, dried thyme, and ½ tsp cayenne and salt. Keeps for 3 months in airtight container.

Grilled TLT Sandwich

A vegetarian version of the diner classic. The longer the tofu marinates the more flavourful it will be.

2 tbsp	tomato paste
2 tbsp	apple cider vinegar
2 tbsp	soy sauce
2 tbsp	water
1 clove	garlic, minced
1 tsp	Splenda
½ tsp	Worcestershire sauce
1 pkg (1 lb)	extra-firm tofu, drained and rinsed
4	large whole wheat tortillas
4	lettuce leaves
1	tomato, sliced

1. In bowl, stir together tomato paste, vinegar, soy sauce, water, garlic, Splenda and Worcestershire sauce. Slice tofu into ½-inch strips and place in baking dish. Pour sauce over and toss to coat well. Cover and marinate in refrigerator for 2 hours or up to 1 day.
2. Preheat oiled grill to medium or oven to 375°F.
3. Remove tofu from marinade and grill strips for 2 minutes per side or leave in baking dish and bake for 20 minutes or until hot.
4. Divide tofu among tortillas. Top with lettuce and tomato slices and roll up.

Makes 4 servings.

Grilled Portobello Mushroom Pizzas

Look for the largest mushrooms you can find. Use any favourite green-light toppings and add chopped cooked lean ham, chicken or turkey for meat lovers.

8	large portobello mushrooms, stems removed
2 tsp	olive oil
½ cup	tomato sauce
½ cup	mozzarella cheese (part skim)

Optional toppings:

Red or green peppers, seeded and chopped

Olives

Chopped fresh basil or oregano

Chopped tomatoes

Minced garlic

1. Preheat oiled grill to medium-high.
2. Brush both sides of mushrooms with oil. Grill mushrooms, stem side down, for 4 minutes. Turn and grill for another 4 minutes or until slightly softened.
3. Top mushrooms with tomato sauce and desired toppings. Sprinkle cheese over top and grill, covered, for 5 minutes or until cheese is bubbling.

Makes 4 main-course or 8 appetizer servings.

Broccoli, Sun-Dried Tomato and Feta Quiche

Serve this easy crustless quiche warm or cold. It pairs well with a side salad for lunch or a light supper.

1 tsp	non-hydrogenated margarine
¼ cup	fresh whole wheat bread crumbs
1 bunch	broccoli, trimmed and cut into florets
1¼ cups	liquid egg
1 cup	skim milk
¼ tsp each	salt and freshly ground pepper
2 slices	fresh whole-grain bread, cubed
2	green onions, chopped
¼ cup	packed sun-dried tomatoes, rehydrated in 1 cup hot water, drained and chopped
2 oz	light-style feta cheese, crumbled

1. Preheat oven to 350°F. Grease bottom and sides of deep 10-inch pie plate with margarine. Add bread crumbs, tilting to coat bottom and sides evenly.

2. Steam broccoli for 5 minutes or until tender-crisp. Rinse under cold water, drain and chop. Set aside.

3. In large bowl, whisk together egg, milk, salt and pepper. Stir in steamed broccoli, cubed bread, green onions, sun-dried tomatoes and feta. Pour into prepared pan.

4. Bake for 50 to 60 minutes or until light golden, puffed and just set in centre.

Makes 6 servings.

Variations:

Quiche Lorraine: Omit broccoli, sun-dried tomatoes and feta. Stir ¼ cup shredded light-style Swiss cheese and 4 slices back bacon, chopped, into egg mixture before baking.

Caramelized Onion, Roasted Red Pepper and Chèvre: Omit broccoli, sun-dried tomatoes, feta and green onion. In non-stick frying pan, heat 2 tsp oil over medium heat. Cook 3 onions, thinly sliced, for about 30 minutes or until golden brown. Stir into egg mixture along with ½ cup chopped roasted red peppers and 2 oz chèvre, crumbled, before baking.

Smoked Salmon: Omit broccoli, sun-dried tomatoes and feta. Stir 4 oz chopped smoked salmon and 2 tbsp chopped fresh dill into egg mixture before baking.

Indian Vegetable Curry

So many wonderful vegetarian dishes come from India. This one has a smooth mild curry flavour, but you can spike up the heat by using a hot curry paste or powder. Serve this with basmati rice.

1 tbsp	canola oil
2	onions, cut in wedges
3 cloves	garlic, minced
1 tbsp	chopped fresh ginger
1 tbsp	mild curry paste or powder
1 tsp	cumin seeds, crushed
3 cups	vegetable stock (low-fat, low-sodium)
2	red bell peppers, chopped
2 cups	broccoli florets
8 oz	green beans, cut into 1-inch pieces
1	zucchini, chopped
1 can (540 mL)	chickpeas, drained and rinsed
¼ cup	chopped fresh cilantro

1. In large saucepan, heat oil over medium heat. Cook onions, garlic, ginger, curry paste and cumin seeds for 5 minutes or until softened. Add stock and bring to boil. Add peppers, broccoli, beans, zucchini and chickpeas. Cover and simmer for about 15 minutes or until vegetables are tender-crisp. Sprinkle with coriander.

Makes 4 servings.

Fettuccine Primavera

Primavera means "springtime" in Italian, and you can use your favourite spring vegetables, such as asparagus or fiddleheads, in this pasta. Fortunately, you can get peppers, tomatoes and peas year-round, so you can make this dish any time.

¼ cup	extra- virgin olive oil
2 cups	cubed firm tofu
3 cloves	garlic, minced
¼ tsp	red pepper flakes
½ cup	vegetable cocktail juice
2 cups	chopped fresh asparagus or peas
1	red pepper, thinly sliced
1	carrot, thinly sliced
1	yellow zucchini, thinly sliced
6 oz	whole wheat fettuccine or linguine pasta
2	plum tomatoes, chopped
¼ cup	chopped fresh flat-leaf parsley
2 tbsp	grated Parmesan cheese

1. In non-stick frying pan, heat 2 tbsp of the oil over medium-high heat. Brown tofu on all sides for about 2 minutes; remove to plate. Reserve oil.

2. In large shallow saucepan, heat remaining oil and reserved oil over medium heat. Cook garlic and red pepper flakes for 1 minute. Add vegetable cocktail juice; bring to boil. Reduce heat and simmer for 1 minute. Add asparagus, red pepper, carrot and zucchini; cook, stirring, for 10 minutes or until vegetables are tender-crisp.

3. Meanwhile, in large pot of boiling salted water, cook fettuccine for 8 minutes or until al dente. Drain and return to pot. Add vegetables and tofu, and toss to coat. Stir in tomatoes, parsley and Parmesan cheese.

Makes 4 servings.

Vegetarian Moussaka

Traditionally made with ground lamb, moussaka can be made green-light by using vegetables.

2	large eggplants (about 3 lbs total)
2 tsp	salt
1 tsp	canola oil
2	large onions, finely chopped
3 cloves	garlic, minced
1 each	red and green pepper, diced
1 tbsp	dried oregano
1 tsp	ground cinnamon
½ tsp	freshly ground pepper
¼ tsp	ground allspice
1 can (796 mL)	diced tomatoes
¼ cup	tomato paste
1 can (540 mL)	chickpeas, drained and rinsed
¼ cup	chopped fresh flat-leaf parsley

Cheese Sauce:

2 tbsp	canola oil
¼ cup	whole wheat flour
2 cups	warm skim milk
¼ tsp	salt
Pinch each	ground nutmeg and freshly ground pepper
⅔ cup	liquid egg
½ cup	1% pressed cottage cheese
1 cup	crumbled light feta cheese

1. Preheat oven to 425°F.

2. Cut eggplants into ¼-inch-thick slices and layer in a colander, sprinkling each layer with some of the salt. Let stand for 30 minutes, then rinse slices and drain well. Place on baking sheets lined with parchment paper and roast, in batches if necessary, for about 20 minutes or until tender. Set aside. Reduce oven temperature to 350°F.

3. In a large, shallow Dutch oven or deep non-stick frying pan, heat oil over medium heat. Cook onions, garlic, red and green peppers, oregano, cinnamon, pepper and allspice until onions have softened, about 5 minutes. Add tomatoes and tomato paste; bring to boil. Add chickpeas and parsley, reduce heat and simmer for 15 minutes.

4. Cheese Sauce: In a saucepan, heat oil over medium heat. Stir in flour and cook for 1 minute. Whisk in milk and cook, whisking gently, for about 10 minutes or until mixture is thick enough to coat the back of a spoon. Stir in salt, nutmeg and pepper. Let cool slightly and whisk in liquid egg and cottage cheese.

5. Spread one-third of the tomato sauce in the bottom of a 13- x 9-inch baking dish. Top with one-third of the eggplant slices and one-quarter of the feta cheese. Repeat the layers. After the last layer of eggplant, spread the cheese sauce evenly over the top and sprinkle with the remaining feta.

6. Bake for about 1 hour or until top is golden brown. Let stand for 10 minutes before serving.

Makes 8 servings.

FISH AND SEAFOOD

Citrus-Poached Haddock

Citrus fruits and fish are made for each other. This simple dish is impressive enough for company.

1	small onion, finely chopped
1 clove	garlic, minced
¼ cup	orange juice
¼ cup	dry white wine or vermouth
1 tbsp	lemon juice
1 tsp	grated lemon zest
¼ cup	fish, chicken or vegetable stock (low-fat, low-sodium)
1 lb	haddock fillet, cut into 4 pieces
2 tbsp	chopped fresh parsley or dill
¼ tsp each	salt and freshly ground pepper

1. In large frying pan, bring onion, garlic, orange juice, wine, lemon juice and zest to boil. Boil until onion is softened and liquid is reduced by half, about 5 minutes.

2. Add stock and return to boil. Place haddock in frying pan; reduce heat and simmer gently, covered, for 10 minutes or until fish flakes easily with a fork. Using slotted spoon, remove haddock to platter and cover with foil to keep warm.

3. Bring poaching liquid to boil and reduce by one-third. Stir in parsley and season with salt and pepper. Pour sauce over fish.

Makes 4 servings.

Miso-Crusted Salmon

This recipe is a quick way to dress up salmon. Leftovers are great cold.

1 clove	garlic, minced
2 tbsp	white miso
1 tbsp	tahini
2 tsp	rice vinegar
1 tsp	mirin or sweet sherry
1 lb	salmon fillet

1. Preheat oven to 425°F.
2. In small bowl, whisk together garlic, miso, tahini, vinegar and mirin.
3. Spread miso mixture evenly over surface of salmon. Bake for 10 to 12 minutes or until salmon flakes easily with a fork.

Makes 4 servings.

Lemon Linguine with Smoked Salmon

This pasta is good even at room temperature. Try it with different vegetables, such as snow peas, edamame or broccoli florets.

¼ cup	lemon juice
1 tbsp	grated lemon zest
2 tbsp	olive oil
¼ tsp	freshly ground pepper
6 oz	whole wheat linguine
¾ cup	fresh or frozen peas
6 oz	smoked salmon, chopped
2	green onions, chopped
¼ cup	chopped fresh parsley

1. In large bowl, whisk together lemon juice and zest, oil and pepper.

2. In large pot of boiling salted water, cook linguine for 5 minutes. Add peas and continue to cook for another 3 minutes or until pasta is al dente. Drain and add to bowl with lemon mixture. Add salmon, green onions and parsley; toss to combine.

Makes 4 servings.

Thai Red Curry Shrimp Pasta

The combination of curry spices, lime and cilantro are hallmarks of Thai cooking.

1 lb	large raw shrimp, peeled and deveined
1 tsp	Thai red curry paste
1 tbsp	extra-virgin olive oil
4 cloves	garlic, minced
2	large tomatoes, peeled, seeded and chopped
¾ cup	dry white wine
	zest and juice of 1 lime
¼ tsp each	salt and freshly ground pepper
2 tbsp	chopped fresh cilantro
6 oz	whole wheat spaghettini or linguine
	lime wedges

1. In bowl, toss shrimp with curry paste until well coated. Cover and refrigerate for at least 2 hours or up to 8 hours.

2. In large non-stick frying pan, heat oil over medium heat. Cook garlic just until starting to turn golden, 1 to 2 minutes. Add tomatoes, wine, lime zest and juice, salt and pepper; bring to boil. Reduce heat and simmer until sauce reduces and thickens, about 8 minutes. Add shrimp and cook, stirring, until pink and firm, 3 to 4 minutes. Stir in cilantro.

3. Meanwhile, in large pot of boiling salted water, cook pasta until al dente, about 8 minutes. Drain and add pasta to shrimp mixture. Toss to coat with sauce. Serve with lime wedges.

Makes 4 servings.

G.I. Fish Fillet

You can use virtually any fish in this simple recipe; salmon and trout are favourites in our house. This makes 1 serving, but you can multiply portions as necessary.

4 oz	fish fillet
1 to 2 tsp	fresh lemon juice
pinch	freshly ground pepper

1. Place fish fillet in microwave-safe dish and sprinkle with lemon juice and pepper. Cover dish with microwave-safe plastic wrap, folding back one corner lightly to allow steam to escape.
2. Microwave on High until fish is opaque and easily flakes with a fork, 4 to 5 minutes. Let stand for 2 minutes, then serve.

Makes 1 serving.

Ginger Wasabi Halibut

This fish can also be cooked on the barbecue. Serve it with Cold Noodle Salad with Cucumber and Sesame (see recipe, page 214) for a refreshing meal.

2 tbsp	Dijon mustard
2 tsp	wasabi powder
3 tbsp	mirin or sweet sherry
2 tbsp	minced ginger root
2 tbsp	chopped fresh cilantro
1 lb	halibut, cut into 4 pieces

1. Preheat oven to 350°F.
2. In bowl, stir together mustard and wasabi powder. Stir in mirin, ginger and cilantro. Place fish in marinade and turn to coat. Let stand at room temperature for 20 minutes.
3. Place halibut on baking sheet and bake for 8 to 10 minutes or until firm to the touch.

Makes 4 servings.

POULTRY

Chicken Tikka

This recipe uses garam masala, an Indian spice mixture with myriad uses.

> $\frac{1}{2}$ cup yogurt cheese (see method below)
> 2 cloves garlic, minced
> 1 tbsp minced fresh ginger
> 2 tsp lemon juice
> 1 tsp salt
> $\frac{1}{2}$ tsp ground cumin
> $\frac{1}{2}$ tsp chili powder
> $\frac{1}{2}$ tsp garam masala
> $\frac{1}{4}$ tsp turmeric
> 1 lb boneless skinless chicken breasts, cut into bite-sized cubes

1. In bowl, stir together yogurt cheese, garlic, ginger, lemon juice, salt, cumin, chili powder, garam masala and turmeric. Add chicken and toss to coat thoroughly with mixture. Cover and marinate in refrigerator for 4 to 6 hours.

2. Preheat oiled grill to medium-high or oven to 400°F.

3. Remove chicken from marinade and thread onto 4 bamboo skewers that have been soaked for 30 minutes.

4. Grill, turning occasionally, until chicken is no longer pink inside, about 10 minutes, or place on baking sheet and bake for 10 to 12 minutes.

Makes 4 servings.

YOGURT CHEESE

Looking for a green-light alternative to sour cream? Try yogurt cheese—it's easy to make your own from plain non-fat yogurt. Place a sieve lined with cheesecloth, paper towels or a coffee filter over a bowl. Spoon the yogurt into the sieve and cover it with plastic wrap. Place the sieve and bowl in the refrigerator. Let the yogurt drain overnight—the next day you will have yogurt cheese.

Chicken Stir-Fry with Broccoli

This quick chicken stir-fry will get everyone eating their broccoli.

1	egg white
1 tsp	Chinese Spice Mix, optional
1 lb	boneless skinless chicken breasts, cut into bite-sized pieces
3 tbsp	orange juice
2 tbsp	soy sauce (low-sodium)
1 tbsp	hoisin sauce
1 tbsp	oyster sauce
2 tsp	cornstarch
1 tsp	sesame oil
1 tbsp	canola oil
2 cloves	garlic, minced
1	onion, thinly sliced
1	red pepper, seeded and sliced
1 tbsp	minced fresh ginger
1	bunch broccoli, trimmed and cut into 1-inch pieces
¼ cup	water
1 cup	bean sprouts
½ cup	coarsely chopped cashews

1. In medium bowl, whisk egg white and spice mix. Add chicken and toss.

2. In small bowl, stir orange juice, soy sauce, hoisin sauce, oyster sauce, cornstarch and sesame oil until smooth. Set aside.

3. In wok or large non-stick frying pan, heat canola oil over high heat. Add chicken mixture and stir-fry for 5 minutes. Remove to plate or bowl.

4. Add garlic, onion, red pepper and ginger. Stir-fry for 1 minute. Add broccoli and water and bring to boil. Cover and cook for 5 minutes or just until broccoli is tender-crisp.

5. Add chicken and sauce, and stir-fry for 3 min. Stir in sprouts and cashews.

White Chicken Chili

This is a quick one-pot meal, perfect for the weekday rush.

2 tsp	olive oil
4 cups	shredded cabbage
3 cloves	garlic, minced
2	onions, chopped
1	carrot, chopped
1	jalapeño pepper, minced (optional)
1 lb	boneless skinless chicken breasts, cubed
2 ½ cups	chicken stock (low-fat, low-sodium)
1 can (19 oz)	cannellini (white kidney) beans, drained and rinsed
2 tsp	ground cumin
1 tsp	chili powder
1 tsp	dried oregano
¼ tsp	salt

Optional toppings:

Salsa, no added sugar
Chopped cilantro
Non-fat sour cream or low-fat plain yogurt

1. In deep frying pan or Dutch oven, heat oil over medium-high heat. Cook cabbage, garlic, onion, carrot and jalapeño pepper, if using, for 10 minutes or until softened, stirring occasionally. Push vegetables to side of pan; add chicken and cook for 3 minutes. Stir in stock, beans, cumin, chili powder, oregano and salt. Cook for 15 to 20 minutes or until chicken is no longer pink inside.

2. Serve with any of the optional toppings over cooked basmati rice, if desired.

Makes 4 to 6 servings.

Chicken Schnitzel

Kids love this dish. You can substitute more traditional veal scaloppine for the chicken.

4	boneless skinless chicken breasts (4 oz each)
½ cup	whole wheat flour
½ tsp each	salt and freshly ground pepper
2	omega-3 egg whites
½ cup	wheat bran
¼ cup	wheat germ
¼ cup	fine dry whole wheat bread crumbs
1 tsp	grated orange zest
1 tbsp	extra-virgin olive oil
½ cup	fresh orange juice
½ cup	chicken stock (low-fat, low-sodium)
½ cup	thinly sliced dried apricots
¼ cup	chopped green onion

1. Using meat mallet or rolling pin, pound chicken breasts between 2 pieces of plastic wrap until about ¼ inch thick.

2. In large, shallow dish or pie plate, combine flour, salt and pepper. In another shallow dish or pie plate, whisk egg whites. In third dish or pie plate, combine bran, wheat germ, bread crumbs and orange zest.

3. Pat chicken dry and dredge in flour mixture, shaking off excess. Dip in egg whites, letting excess drip off, then dredge in bran mixture, coating completely.

4. In large non-stick frying pan, heat oil over medium- high heat. Fry chicken (in batches, if necessary) for 4 minutes per side or until golden brown and just cooked through. Transfer schnitzel to platter and place in 200°F oven to keep warm.

5. In same frying pan, combine orange juice, stock and apricots. Bring to boil and reduce until slightly thickened and syrupy, about 3 minutes. Stir in green onion. Pour sauce over schnitzel.

Makes 4 servings.

Orange Chicken With Almonds

Fans of sweet-and-sour dishes will enjoy this orange-flavoured chicken. The almonds add calcium. Serve over basmati rice.

2	oranges
1 tbsp	canola oil
2	boneless skinless chicken breasts (4 oz each), diced
2 tsp	minced ginger root
¼ tsp each	salt and freshly ground pepper
2	green onions, chopped
1 each	red and green pepper, chopped
Pinch	red pepper flakes
¼ cup	chicken stock (low-fat, low-sodium)
3 tbsp	soy sauce (low-sodium)
2 tsp	cornstarch
½ cup	sliced almonds, toasted

1. Using rasp or grater, remove 1 tsp of the orange zest and set aside. Cut away orange zest and pith from one of the oranges and discard. Chop orange flesh coarsely. Cut other orange in half and squeeze out juice; set aside, discarding rind.

2. In large non-stick frying pan or wok, heat 1 ½ tsp of the oil over medium-high heat. Cook chicken, ginger and a pinch each of the salt and pepper for about 6 minutes per side or until chicken is no longer pink inside. Transfer to plate. Add remaining oil to frying pan and cook green onions, red and green pepper, and red pepper flakes, stirring constantly, for about 6 minutes or until tender-crisp.

3. In small bowl, whisk together chicken stock, soy sauce, reserved orange zest and juice, cornstarch and remaining salt and pepper. Add chicken, chopped orange and vegetable mixture to frying pan and cook, stirring, for about 5 minutes or until sauce is thickened and chicken and vegetables are coated. Sprinkle with almonds and serve with rice.

Makes 2 servings.

Chicken Tarragon with Mushrooms

Tarragon adds a light French flavour. The dish below is great for entertaining.

2 tsp	canola oil
2	boneless skinless chicken breasts (4 oz each)
½ tsp	freshly ground pepper
1 tsp	non-hydrogenated soft margarine
1	small onion, chopped
8 oz	mushrooms, sliced
3 tbsp	vermouth or white wine
1 tbsp	chopped fresh tarragon
½ cup	chicken stock (low-fat, low-sodium) or water

1. In non-stick frying pan, heat oil over medium-high heat. Sprinkle chicken with pepper and cook for about 6 minutes per side or until no longer pink inside. Transfer to plate and cover to keep warm.

2. Add margarine to frying pan and cook onion and mushrooms, stirring constantly, until soft, about 5 minutes. Add vermouth and tarragon, and simmer for 1 minute. Add stock and simmer for 2 minutes or until reduced by half. Season with pepper.

3. Serve sauce over chicken.

Makes 2 servings.

Spicy Roasted Chicken with Tomatoes and Tarragon

This recipe is also from our friend Meryle. Serve it with basmati rice or quinoa to soak up the sauce.

4 cups	cherry or grape tomatoes, halved
5 cloves	garlic, crushed
¼ cup	extra-virgin olive oil
2 tbsp	chopped fresh tarragon
2 tsp	red pepper flakes
4	boneless skinless chicken breasts (4 oz each)
1 tsp each	salt and freshly ground pepper

1. Preheat oven to 450°F.

2. In large bowl, toss tomatoes with garlic, oil, 1 tbsp of the tarragon, and red pepper flakes.

3. Place chicken on rimmed baking sheet. Arrange tomato mixture in single layer around chicken. Sprinkle chicken and tomato mixture with salt and pepper. Roast for 30 to 35 minutes or until chicken is no longer pink inside. Transfer chicken to platter. Spoon tomatoes and juices over chicken and sprinkle with remaining tarragon.

Makes 4 servings.

Zesty Barbecued Chicken

The marinade in this recipe helps keep the breasts moist when they are cooked.

¼ cup	lemon juice
2 tsp	chopped fresh rosemary
2 tsp	canola oil
4	boneless skinless chicken breasts (4 oz each)
⅓ cup	Zesty Barbecue Sauce (see recipe, page 247)

1. In bowl, whisk together lemon juice, rosemary and oil. Add chicken breasts; toss to coat. Marinate at room temperature for 30 minutes.

2. Meanwhile, preheat oiled grill to medium-high.

3. Remove chicken from marinade and discard marinade. Brush chicken with Zesty Barbecue Sauce; grill for 6 minutes. Turn, brush with more sauce and grill for another 6 minutes or until chicken is no longer pink inside.

Makes 4 servings.

Zesty Barbecue Sauce

This sauce will keep up to 2 weeks refrigerated in an airtight container.

1 can (398 mL)	tomato sauce
2 cloves	garlic, minced
¼ cup	frozen apple juice concentrate
¼ cup	tomato paste
2 tbsp	cider vinegar
1 tbsp	Splenda
1 tbsp	Dijon mustard
2 tsp	chili powder
½ tsp	Worcestershire sauce
¼ tsp each	salt and freshly ground pepper

1. In large saucepan, combine tomato sauce, garlic, apple juice concentrate, tomato paste, vinegar, Splenda, mustard, chili powder, Worcestershire sauce, salt and pepper; bring to boil. Reduce heat and simmer, uncovered, for about 20 minutes or until reduced and thickened.

Makes about 1 ½ cups.

MEAT

Stuffed Peppers

Here's a twist on a classic comfort dish.

12 oz	extra-lean ground beef
2 cloves	garlic, minced
1	onion, chopped
1	omega-3 egg
¾ cup	barley
2 tbsp	tomato paste
½ tsp each	salt and freshly ground pepper
4	large peppers (any colour)
2 cups	Basic Tomato Sauce

1. In bowl, mix together beef, garlic, onion, egg, barley, tomato paste, salt and pepper.

2. Cut top off each pepper and remove seeds and ribs. Pack each with beef mixture. Place in large saucepan and add enough water to just cover top of peppers. (Don't worry if they turn on their sides during cooking; the filling will stay put.) Bring to boil; reduce heat and simmer for 45 minutes or until barley is tender. Remove peppers from water and place on serving platter. Heat tomato sauce and pour over peppers before serving.

Makes 4 servings.

Make Ahead: Peppers can be prepared up to 1 day ahead; cover and refrigerate. Or wrap well and freeze up to 1 month. Microwave from frozen, or thaw in refrigerator and reheat in oven. Pour hot tomato sauce over reheated peppers.

Meatloaf

Extra-lean ground beef is still relatively high in fat. For this meatloaf, a lower-fat and better alternative to ground beef is an equal amount of ground turkey or chicken breast.

1 ½ lbs	extra-lean ground beef
1 cup	tomato juice
½ cup	large-flake rolled oats (uncooked)
1	omega-3 egg, lightly beaten
½ cup	chopped onion
1 tbsp	Worcestershire sauce
½ tsp	salt (optional)
¼ tsp	freshly ground pepper

1. Preheat oven to 350°F.
2. In large bowl, combine beef, tomato juice, oats, egg, onion, Worcestershire sauce, salt (if using) and pepper. Mix lightly but thoroughly.
3. Press meatloaf mixture into an 8- × 4-inch loaf pan. Bake for 1 hour, or until an instant-read meat thermometer inserted into the centre registers 160°F. Let meatloaf stand for 5 minutes before draining off any juices and slicing.

Makes 6 servings.

Beef Cutlets in Mushroom Gravy

An updated version of old-fashioned Salisbury steak. The beef stays moist and juicy while cooking in the beefy gravy. Serve with new potatoes and green beans for a comforting supper.

1	omega-3 egg
2 cloves	garlic, minced
1/3 cup	crushed whole wheat crackers
1/3 cup	chopped black or green olives
1/2 cup	grated carrot
1 tsp	Worcestershire sauce
1/4 tsp	salt
1/2 tsp	freshly ground pepper
12 oz	extra-lean ground beef
2 tsp	olive oil
1	large onion, sliced
8 oz	mushrooms, sliced
2 cups	beef broth (low-fat, low-sodium)
1 tbsp	tomato paste

1. In large bowl, whisk egg. Add garlic, crackers, olives, carrot, Worcestershire sauce, salt and pepper; stir to combine. Add ground beef and combine well, using hands to distribute ingredients evenly.

2. Preheat oiled grill to medium-high.

3. Form meat mixture into 4 oval patties, each about 3/4-inch thick. Place on grill or in non-stick frying pan and cook until browned, 3 to 4 minutes per side.

4. Meanwhile, heat oil in large non-stick frying pan over medium-high heat. Cook onion and mushrooms until softened and turning golden, about 8 minutes. Stir in broth and tomato paste; bring to boil. Add beef cutlets, cover and simmer for 10 minutes or until beef is no longer pink inside.

Makes 4 servings.

Blueberry Beef Burgers

Blueberries help make these burgers moist and juicy.

½ cup	fresh or frozen and thawed wild blueberries
2 cloves	garlic, minced
1 tbsp	balsamic vinegar
1 tbsp	Dijon mustard
1 tsp	Worcestershire sauce
½ tsp	salt
¼ tsp	freshly ground pepper
½ cup	ground flaxseed
¼ cup	rolled oats
1 lb	extra-lean ground beef
2	whole wheat buns
4	lettuce leaves
4	tomato slices

1. Preheat oiled grill or broiler to medium-high.

2. Place blueberries in bowl of food processor. Add garlic, vinegar, mustard, Worcestershire sauce, salt and pepper; purée. Scrape into large bowl. Stir in flaxseed and oats. Add ground beef and mix with hands or wooden spoon until well combined.

3. Form meat mixture into 4 patties, each about ½-inch thick. Place on grill or broiler pan and cook, turning once, until no longer pink inside, 4 to 5 minutes per side. Serve each patty on half a whole wheat bun. Top with lettuce and tomato slices.

Makes 4 servings.

Bolognese Pasta Sauce

This is a great staple sauce to have on hand. Freeze it in 1-cup portions in zip-top plastic freezer bags and place in the fridge overnight to defrost. Use in lasagna, serve with whole wheat pasta combined with cooked kidney beans, or serve over brown basmati rice.

1 tbsp	olive oil
1 lb	extra-lean ground beef
½ cup	skim milk
2 cloves	garlic, minced
1	onion, chopped
1	red pepper, seeded and chopped
1	green pepper, seeded and chopped
1 stalk	celery, chopped
1	carrot, chopped
1 tbsp	dried oregano
1 tsp	salt
½ tsp	freshly ground pepper
1 cup	red wine or unsweetened pure grape juice
2 cans (28 oz each)	crushed tomatoes
1 tbsp	chopped fresh basil

1. In large pot or deep frying pan, heat oil over medium-high heat. Cook beef for about 8 minutes or until browned. Pour in milk and cook for another 2 to 3 minutes or until milk is absorbed. Reduce heat to medium. Add garlic, onion, red and green peppers, celery, carrot, oregano, salt and pepper; cook, stirring, for about 5 minutes or until vegetables are softened. Pour in wine and cook, stirring and scraping up any brown bits, for about 1 minute or until wine is evaporated.

2. Add tomatoes and basil; bring to boil. Reduce heat and simmer, uncovered, for about 45 minutes or until sauce is thick and flavourful.

Makes about 6 cups.

Pork Medallions Dijon

Eating the green-light way doesn't mean you have to sacrifice flavour. This pork is fork-tender, and the tasty sauce is rich and creamy.

2	pork tenderloins (about 12 oz each)
5 tbsp	whole wheat flour
¾ tsp each	salt and freshly ground pepper
2 tbsp	extra-virgin olive oil
2	onions, thinly sliced
1 clove	garlic, minced
¼ cup	Dijon mustard
1 ¼ cups	skim milk
½ cup	dry white wine
1 tbsp	chopped fresh tarragon

1. Slice pork into ¾-inch medallions. Place between 2 pieces of waxed paper; using meat mallet or rolling pin, pound to about ¼-inch thickness.

2. On dinner plate, combine 3 tbsp of the flour and ½ tsp each of the salt and pepper; dredge pork. In large non-stick frying pan, heat 1 tbsp of the oil over medium-high heat. Cook pork until golden brown on both sides, 5 to 7 minutes; transfer to the plate and cover to keep warm.

3. In same frying pan, heat remaining oil over medium heat. Cook onions and garlic, stirring often, for 5 minutes or until softened. Reduce heat to medium-low; cook, stirring occasionally, for 10 minutes or until golden. Add remaining flour and stir to coat onion. Add mustard; cook for 2 minutes. Stir in milk, wine and remaining salt and pepper. Cook, stirring constantly, until thickened. (If mixture is too thick, stir in 1 tbsp warm water.) Stir in tarragon. Return pork to pan and cook until heated through, about 1 minute.

Makes 6 servings.

SNACKS

Crunchy Chickpeas

This is an addictive snack with all the crunch and saltiness of chips and pretzels but without the fat! Experiment with other spices to change the flavour.

2 cans (540 mL each)	chickpeas, drained and rinsed
2 tbsp	extra-virgin olive oil or canola oil
½ tsp	salt
Pinch	cayenne pepper

1. Preheat oven to 400° F.
2. In large bowl, toss chickpeas with oil, salt and cayenne. Spread on large baking sheet in a single layer.
3. Bake for about 45 minutes or until golden, shaking pan a couple of times during cooking. Let cool completely.

Makes 6 servings.

Cranberry Cinnamon Bran Muffins

These muffins are very nutritious with a high fibre content and have a great cinnamon flavour. They can be kept at room temperature for about 2 days or frozen for up to 1 month. (Wrap each muffin individually before freezing to help prevent freezer burn. Then place them in a resealable plastic bag or airtight container.)

1 cup	wheat bran
½ cup	All-Bran or 100% Bran cereal
¼ tsp	salt
½ cup	boiling water
1 cup	skim milk
1 cup	dried cranberries
⅓ cup	Splenda
1	omega-3 egg
¼ cup	canola oil
1 ¼ cups	whole wheat flour
1 ¼ tsp	baking soda
1 tsp	ground cinnamon

1. Preheat oven to 375°F. Line a 12-cup muffin tin with paper or foil liners.
2. In bowl, combine bran, cereal and salt. Pour boiling water over and stir to combine. Stir in milk and cranberries and set aside.
3. In another bowl, whisk together Splenda, egg and oil. Stir into bran mixture.
4. In large bowl, stir together flour, baking soda and cinnamon. Pour bran mixture over flour mixture and stir until just combined.
5. Divide batter among muffin cups. Bake for about 20 minutes or until tester inserted in centre of muffin comes out clean.

Makes 12 muffins.

Banana Bread

Spread a slice of this quick bread with a teaspoon of light cream cheese.

1½ cups	whole wheat flour
¾ cup	ground flaxseed
2 tsp	baking powder
1 tsp	baking soda
1 tsp	cinnamon
½ tsp	salt
1 cup	mashed very ripe banana (about 3)
¾ cup	Splenda
¾ cup	buttermilk
½ cup	liquid egg
1 tsp	vanilla

1. Preheat oven to 350°F. Oil a 9- by 5-inch loaf pan.
2. In bowl, stir together flour, flaxseed, baking powder, baking soda, cinnamon and salt.
3. In another bowl, mix together banana, Splenda, buttermilk, egg and vanilla. Pour into flour mixture and stir just until moistened.
4. Pour batter into prepared pan. Bake for 45 to 50 minutes or until tester inserted in centre comes out clean. Let cool on rack.

Makes 1 loaf.

Make Ahead: Wrap in plastic wrap or foil and store at room temperature up to 3 days or freeze up to 1 month.

Apple Bran Muffins

Ruth created this recipe several years ago when I was trying to lose weight. We would make large batches and freeze them. Then, whenever I needed a snack, I'd warm one in the microwave. They were so convenient and delicious.

³⁄₄ cup	All-Bran or Bran Buds cereal
1 cup	skim milk
²⁄₃ cup	whole wheat flour
¹⁄₃ cup	Splenda
2 tsp	baking powder
¹⁄₂ tsp	baking soda
¹⁄₄ tsp	salt
1 tsp	ground allspice
¹⁄₂ tsp	ground cloves
1 ¹⁄₄ cups	oat bran
²⁄₃ cup	raisins
1	large apple, peeled and cut into ¹⁄₄-inch cubes
1	omega-3 egg, lightly beaten
2 tsp	canola oil
¹⁄₂ cup	unsweetened applesauce

1. Preheat oven to 350°F. Line a 12-cup muffin tin with paper or foil liners.

2. In a bowl, combine cereal and milk; let stand for a few minutes.

3. In large bowl, stir together flour, Splenda, baking powder, baking soda, salt, allspice and cloves. Stir in oat bran, raisins and apple.

4. In small bowl, combine egg, oil and applesauce. Stir, along with cereal mixture, into dry ingredients.

5. Divide batter among muffin cups. Bake until lightly browned, about 20 minutes.

Makes 12 muffins.

Whole Wheat Fruit Scones

Enjoy these scones with a hot cup of tea. They are even better with a little sugar-free fruit spread.

1 ½ cups	whole wheat flour
½ cup	oat bran
½ cup	chopped dried apricots or dried cranberries
2 tbsp	Splenda
2 tsp	baking powder
½ tsp	salt
¼ tsp	ground nutmeg
¼ cup	non- hydrogenated soft margarine
⅔ cup	skim milk
2 tbsp	liquid egg

1. Preheat oven to 425°F.

2. In large bowl, combine flour, oat bran, dried apricots, Splenda, baking powder, salt and nutmeg. Using your fingers, rub margarine into flour mixture to combine. Add milk and toss with fork to form soft dough.

3. Place dough on floured surface and knead gently about 5 times. Pat dough out to ½-inch thickness. Cut dough into 8 squares, or use cookie or biscuit cutter to cut scones.

4. Place on baking sheet and brush tops with liquid egg. Bake for about 12 minutes or until golden on bottom.

Makes 8 scones.

Strawberry Tea Bread

This recipe makes two loaves, one for now and one for the freezer (wrap in foil and plastic wrap and freeze up to 1 month.) A slice makes a perfect snack or a delicious dessert paired with sliced berries.

1 ½ cups	whole wheat flour
1 ½ cups	rolled oats
½ cup	wheat bran
1 tsp	cinnamon
1 tsp	baking soda
½ tsp	baking powder
½ tsp	salt
¾ cup	liquid egg
¾ cup	Splenda
½ cup	canola oil
½ cup	skim milk
1 tsp	vanilla
4 cups	strawberries, fresh or frozen and thawed, mashed

1. Preheat oven to 375°F. Oil two 9- × 5-inch loaf pans.

2. In large bowl, stir together flour, oats, bran, cinnamon, baking soda, baking powder and salt; set aside.

3. In separate bowl, whisk together liquid egg, Splenda, oil, milk and vanilla. Pour over dry ingredients and stir just until moistened. Stir in strawberries.

4. Divide mixture evenly between pans. Bake for 45 to 50 minutes or until cake tester inserted in centre comes out clean. Let cool in pan on rack for 15 minutes. Turn out onto rack and let cool completely.

Makes 2 loaves, 14 to 16 slices each. One serving is 1 slice.

DESSERTS

Creamy Raspberry Mousse

No one will know this dessert is so easy to make. Serve it as is or dress it up with some fresh fruit or berries.

1 cup	cottage cheese (1%)
1 cup	frozen raspberries
2 tbsp	Splenda
1 tbsp	amaretto or berry-flavoured liqueur (optional)

1. Combine all ingredients in a food processor and process until smooth. Serve immediately or refrigerate in airtight container for up to 3 days.

Makes 4 servings

Fancy Fruit Salad

Use pretty glass serving dishes and layer fruit for effect. Vary the fruit combination for colour and taste.

1 pint	strawberries sliced (keep 4 whole for top)
1 pint	fresh berries (blueberries, blackberries)
2 tbsp	orange juice
½ tsp	ground cinnamon
¼ tsp	ground nutmeg
1 tsp	Splenda (or more to taste)
4	kiwi peeled and sliced
4	sprigs of mint (optional)

1. Wash and drain fruit. Sprinkle berries with sugar substitute.
2. Combine together the orange juice and nutmeg in a small bowl. Layer fruits in dish, ending with slices of kiwi on top.
3. Drizzle each dish with a small amount of orange juice mixture. Top with whole strawberry and mint if using. Serve with sweetened strained yogurt on the side.

Berry Crumble

This is one of Ruth's favourite green-light desserts. Though it's best made with fresh berries during the summer, it's also lovely with frozen fruit.

5 cups	fresh or frozen berries, such as raspberries, blackberries, blueberries and sliced strawberries
1	large apple, cored and chopped
2 tbsp	whole wheat flour
2 tbsp	Splenda
½ tsp	ground cinnamon

Topping:

1 cup	large-flake oats
½ cup	chopped pecans or walnuts
¼ cup	brown Splenda
¼ cup	non-hydrogenated soft margarine, melted
1 tsp	ground cinnamon

1. Preheat oven to 350°F.
2. In 8-inch square baking dish, combine berries and apple.
3. In bowl, combine flour, Splenda and cinnamon. Sprinkle over fruit and toss gently.
4. In medium bowl, combine oats, pecans, brown Splenda, margarine and cinnamon. Sprinkle over fruit mixture. Bake for about 30 minutes or until fruit is tender and top is golden.

Makes 6 servings.

Variation: Prepare as above and microwave on High for about 6 minutes or until fruit is tender. The top won't get golden or crisp in the microwave.

Rhubarb-Ginger Cobbler

Fresh rhubarb heralds the start of spring, but use frozen rhubarb to enjoy this homey heart-warming dessert year-round.

4 cups	chopped fresh or frozen rhubarb
½ cup	Splenda
2 tbsp	cornstarch
1 tbsp	grated fresh ginger

Topping:

1 cup	whole wheat flour
1 cup	large-flake oats
¼ cup	Splenda
1 tbsp	baking powder
1 tsp	baking soda
¼ tsp	salt
½ cup	liquid egg
½ cup	low-fat plain yogurt
½ cup	skim milk
1 tsp	vanilla

1. Preheat oven to 400°F. Oil an 8-inch square baking pan.

2. In bowl, toss together rhubarb, Splenda, cornstarch and ginger; spoon into prepared pan. Set aside.

3. Topping: In large bowl, combine flour, oats, Splenda, baking powder, baking soda and salt. In small bowl, whisk together egg, yogurt, milk and vanilla. Add to flour mixture and stir until just moistened. Drop topping by spoonfuls over fruit.

4. Bake for 25 to 30 minutes or until topping is golden and filling is bubbly. Let cool slightly before serving.

Makes 6 servings.

Apple Raspberry Coffee Cake

This fruit-laden cake makes a delectable light dessert. It can be refrigerated for up to 3 days.

1 cup	whole wheat flour
½ cup	wheat bran
½ cup	brown Splenda
1 ½ tsp	baking powder
½ tsp	baking soda
¼ tsp	ground cinnamon
¼ tsp	ground nutmeg
Pinch	salt
½ cup	buttermilk
¼ cup	non-hydrogenated soft margarine, melted and cooled
¼ cup	liquid egg
2 tsp	vanilla
1 cup	fresh raspberries
1	apple, cored and diced

Topping:

⅓ cup	large-flake oats
¼ cup	brown Splenda
2 tbsp	chopped pecans
1 tbsp	non-hydrogenated soft margarine

1. Preheat oven to 350°F. Line an 8-inch square baking pan with parchment paper.
2. In large bowl, stir together flour, bran, brown Splenda, baking powder, baking soda, cinnamon, nutmeg and salt; set aside.
3. In another bowl, whisk buttermilk, margarine, liquid egg and vanilla. Stir into flour mixture until moistened. Spread two-thirds of the batter in prepared baking pan.
4. Toss raspberries and apple together and sprinkle over batter. Dollop with remaining batter, smoothly gently with wet spatula.
5. In bowl, combine oats, brown Splenda, pecans and margarine. Sprinkle over top of cake; press gently into batter. Bake for about 30 minutes or until tester inserted in centre comes out clean. Makes 9 servings.

Chocolate Pudding

Ruth loves chocolate and strawberries. This dessert is one of her favourites.

¼ cup	cocoa powder
¼ cup	cornstarch (or 2 tbsp arrowroot)
2 tbsp	Splenda
¼ tsp	salt
2 cups	skim milk
2 tsp	vanilla
1 cup	raspberries or sliced strawberries, or mixture (optional)

1. In saucepan, stir together cocoa, cornstarch, Splenda and salt. Add milk and vanilla and cook over medium-high heat, stirring constantly, until boiling and thickened. Continue cooking, stirring, for 3 minutes. Remove from heat and stir in berries, if using.

2. Pour into serving bowl or 4 individual serving dishes. Let cool to room temperature or place plastic wrap directly on surface and chill in refrigerator before serving.

Makes 4 servings.

Make Ahead: Refrigerate up to 2 days.

Cran-Apple Oatmeal Bars

Tuck these nutritious treats into packed lunches.

3 cups	large-flake oats
1 ½ cups	whole wheat flour
2 tsp	ground cinnamon
1 tsp	baking powder
1 tsp	baking soda
¼ tsp	salt
¾ cup	Splenda
¼ cup	non-hydrogenated margarine (light)
1	omega-3 egg
1	egg white
¾ cup	unsweetened apple sauce
2 tsp	vanilla
1 cup	dried cranberries

1. Preheat oven to 350°F. Line a 13- × 9-inch baking pan with parchment paper.

2. In large bowl, combine oats, whole wheat flour, cinnamon, baking powder, baking soda and salt.

3. In another bowl, beat together Splenda and margarine until fluffy. Beat in egg, egg white, applesauce and vanilla. Add oat mixture and stir to combine. Stir in cranberries. Scrape dough into prepared baking pan and bake for 20 minutes or until cake tester inserted in centre comes out clean. Let cool completely and cut into bars.

Makes 24 bars.

Pecan Brownies

Brownies, you ask? That's right. These are packed with fibre and are absolutely scrumptious, so get baking! Store in an airtight container for up to 4 days or freeze for up to 2 weeks.

1 can (540 mL)	white or red kidney or black beans, drained and rinsed
½ cup	skim milk
⅓ cup	liquid egg
¼ cup	non- hydrogenated soft margarine, melted
1 tbsp	vanilla
¾ cup	Splenda
½ cup	whole wheat flour
½ cup	unsweetened cocoa powder
1 tsp	baking powder
Pinch	salt
½ cup	chopped toasted pecans

1. Preheat oven to 350°F. Line an 8-inch square baking pan with parchment paper.

2. In food processor, purée beans until coarse. Add milk, liquid egg, margarine and vanilla, and purée until smooth, scraping down sides a few times. Set aside.

3. In large bowl, combine Splenda, flour, cocoa, baking powder and salt. Pour bean mixture over flour mixture and stir to combine. Scrape batter into prepared pan, smoothing top. Sprinkle with pecans.

4. Bake for about 18 minutes or until tester inserted in centre comes out clean. Let cool on rack, then cut into 16 squares.

Makes 16 brownies. One serving is one brownie.

Creamy Lemon Squares

These tiny treats make an ideal mid-afternoon pick-me-up. The squares can be stored for up to 3 days or frozen up to 1 month.

½ cup	whole wheat flour
½ cup	wheat bran
½ cup	ground almonds
¼ cup	Splenda
¼ cup	non- hydrogenated soft margarine

Filling:

1 cup	Splenda
¾ cup	liquid egg
2 tsp	grated lemon zest
½ cup	fresh lemon juice
¼ cup	buttermilk
2 tsp	cornstarch
1 tsp	baking powder

1. Preheat oven to 350°F. Oil an 8-inch square baking pan.

2. In mixer or food processor, combine flour, bran, almonds and Splenda. Cut in margarine until mixture is crumbly.

3. Press mixture evenly into bottom of prepared pan. Bake for 20 to 25 minutes or until lightly browned. Set aside to cool, leaving oven on.

4. In bowl, whisk together Splenda and liquid egg. Stir in lemon zest and juice, buttermilk, cornstarch and baking powder. Pour over base. Bake for 15 to 20 minutes or until filling is set. Let cool to room temperature, then refrigerate for at least 2 hours before cutting into squares.

Makes 36 squares. One serving is 2 squares.

APPENDIX
Complete G.I. Diet Food Guide

BEANS

Baked beans with pork	Chili	Baked beans (low-fat)
Broad		Black beans
Refried		Black-eyed peas
		Butter beans
		Cannellini
		Chickpeas/garbanzo
		Italian
		Kidney
		Lentils
		Lima
		Mung
		Navy
		Pigeon
		Refried (low-fat)
		Romano
		Soybeans
		Split peas

BEVERAGES

Alcoholic drinks*	Diet soft drinks	Bottled water
Coconut milk	(caffeinated)	Club soda
Fruit drinks	Milk (1%)	Decaffeinated coffee
Milk (whole or 2%)	Most unsweetened juice	(with skim milk, no
Regular coffee	Red wine*	sugar)
Regular soft drinks	Vegetable juices	Diet soft drinks (no
Rice milk	Coconut milk (low-fat)	caffeine)
Sweetened juice		Herbal tea
Watermelon juice		Light instant chocolate
		Milk (skim)
		Soy milk (plain, low-fat)
		Tea (with skim milk, no
		sugar)

BREADS

Bagels	Crispbreads (with fibre)*	Crispbreads (with high
Baguette/Croissants	Pita (whole wheat)	fibre, e.g., Wasa Fiber)*
Cake/Cookies	Tortillas (whole wheat)	Pita (high-fibre)
Cornbread	Whole-grain breads	Whole-grain, high-fibre
Crispbreads (regular)		breads (min. 3 g fibre
Croutons		per slice)*

* Limit serving size (see page 25).

BREADS

English muffins		
Hamburger buns		
Hot dog buns		
Kaiser rolls		
Melba toast		
Muffins/Doughnuts		
Pancakes/Waffles		
Pizza		
Stuffing		
Tortillas		
White bread		

CEREALS

All cold cereals except those listed as yellow- or green-light	Kashi Good Friends	100% bran
Cereal/Granola bars	Shredded Wheat Bran	All-Bran
Granola		Bran Buds
Grits		Cold cereals with minimum 10 g fibre or protein per serving
Muesli (commercial)		Fibre 1
		Fibre First
		Kashi Go Lean
		Kashi Go Lean Crunch
		Oat Bran
		Porridge (large-flake oats)
		Red River

CEREAL/GRAINS

Amaranth	Cornstarch	Arrowroot flour
Almond flour	Spelt	Barley
Couscous	Whole wheat couscous	Bran (wheat/oat)
Millet		Buckwheat
Polenta		Bulgar
Rice (short-grain, white, instant)		Gram flour
Rice cakes		Kamut
Rice noodles		Kasha (not puffed)
White flour		Quinoa
		Rice (basmati, wild, brown, long-grain)
		Wheat berries
		Wheat germ
		Whole wheat flour

CONDIMENTS/SEASONINGS

BBQ sauce	Mayonnaise (light)	Capers
Croutons		Chili powder
Honey mustard		Extracts (vanilla, etc.)
Ketchup		Garlic
Mayonnaise		Gravy mix (maximum 20
Relish		calories per 1/4 cup
Steak sauce		serving)
Tartar sauce		Herbs
		Horseradish
		Hummus
		Mayonnaise (fat-free)
		Mustard
		Salsa (no added sugar)
		Sauerkraut
		Soy sauce (low-sodium)
		Spices
		Teriyaki sauce
		Vinegar
		Worcestershire sauce

DAIRY

Almond milk	Cheese (low-fat)	Buttermilk
Cheese	Cream cheese (light)	Cottage cheese (1% or
Chocolate milk	Ice cream (low-fat)	fat-free)
Coconut milk	Milk (1%)	Cream cheese (fat-free)
Cottage cheese (whole	Sour cream (light)	Extra-low-fat cheese
or 2%)	Yogurt (low-fat, with	(e.g., Laughing Cow
Cream	sugar)	Light, Boursin Light)
Cream cheese		Frozen yogurt (1/2 cup
Evaporated milk		low-fat)
Goat milk		Flavoured yogurt (non-
Ice cream		fat with sweetener)
Milk (whole or 2%)		Ice cream (1/2 cup, low-fat
Rice milk		and no added sugar)
Sour cream		Milk (skim)
Yogurt (whole or 2%)		Sour cream (1% or less)
		Soy milk (plain, low-fat)
		Soy cheese (low-fat)
		Whey protein powder

FATS AND OILS

Butter	100% nut butters	Almonds*
Coconut oil	100% peanut butter	Canola oil*/seed
Hard margarine	Corn oil	Cashews*
Lard	Mayonnaise (light)	Flax seed
Mayonnaise	Most nuts	Hazelnuts*
Palm oil	Peanuts	Macadamia nuts*
Peanut butter (regular	Pecans	Mayonnaise (fat-free)
and light)	Salad dressings (light)	Olive oil*

* Limit serving size (see page 25).

FATS AND OILS

Salad dressings (regular)	Sesame oil	Pistachios***
Tropical oils	Soft margarine (non-hydrogenated)	Salad dressings (low-fat, low-sugar)
Vegetable shortening	Soy oil	Soft margarine (non-hydrogenated, light)***
	Sunflower oil	
	Vegetable oils	Vegetable oil sprays
	Walnuts	

FRUITS

FRESH/FROZEN	Cantaloupe	Apricots	Apples
	Honeydew melon	Bananas	Avocado***($^1/_4$)
	Kumquats	Custard apples	Blackberries
	Watermelon	Figs	Cherries
		Kiwi	Cranberries
		Mango	Grapefruit
		Papaya	Grapes
		Persimmon	Guavas
		Pineapple	Lemons
		Pomegranates	Nectarines
			Oranges (all varieties)
			Peaches
			Plums
			Pears
			Raspberries
			Rhubarb
			Strawberries
BOTTLED, CANNED and DRIED	All canned fruit in syrup	Canned apricots in juice or water	Applesauce (without sugar)
	Applesauce containing sugar	Dried apricots**	Dried apples
	Most dried fruit** (including dates and raisins)	Dried cranberries**	Fruit spreads with fruit, not sugar as the main ingredient
		Fruit cocktail in juice	
	Prunes	Peaches/pears in syrup	Mandarin oranges
			Peaches/pears in juice or water

JUICES*

*Whenever possible, eat the fruit rather than drink its juice.	Fruit drinks	Apple (unsweetened)	
	Prune	Cranberry (unsweetened)	
	Sweetened juice	Grapefruit (unsweetened)	
	Watermelon	Orange (unsweetened)	
		Pear (unsweetened)	
		Pineapple (unsweetened)	
		Vegetable	

**For baking, it is OK to use a modest amount of dried apricots or cranberries
*** Limit serving size (see page 25).

MEAT, POULTRY, FISH, EGGS AND MEAT SUBSTITUTES

Beef (brisket, short ribs)	Beef* (sirloin steak, sirloin tip)	All fish and seafood, fresh, frozen or canned (in water)
Bologna	Chicken/turkey leg (skinless)	Back bacon
Breaded fish and seafood	Corn beef	Beef (top/eye round steak)
Duck	Dried beef	Chicken breast (skinless)
Goose	Fish canned in oil	Egg whites
Ground beef (more than 10% fat)	Flank steak	Ground beef (extra lean)
Hamburgers	Ground beef (lean)	Lean deli meats
Hot dogs	Lamb (fore/leg shank, centre cut loin chop)	Liquid eggs (e.g., Break Free)
Lamb (rack)	Pork (centre loin, fresh ham, shank, sirloin, top loin)	Moose
Organ meats	Tofu (firm)	Pastrami (turkey)
Pastrami (beef)	Turkey bacon	Pork tenderloin
Pâté	Whole regular eggs (preferably omega-3)	Rabbit
Pork (back ribs, blade, spare ribs)		Sashimi
Regular bacon		Soy/Whey protein powder
Salami		Soy cheese (low-fat)
Sausages		Tofu (soft)
Sushi		Turkey breast (skinless)
		Turkey roll
		TVP (Textured Vegetable Protein)
		Veal
		Veggie burger
		Venison

PASTA*

All canned pastas		Capellini
Gnocchi		Fettucine
Macaroni and cheese		Macaroni
Noodles (canned or instant)		Mung bean noodles
Pasta filled with cheese or meat		Penne
Rice noodles		Rigatoni
		Spaghetti/Linguine
		Vermicelli

PASTA SAUCES

Alfredo	Basil pesto	Light sauces with vegetables (no added sugar, e.g., Healthy Choice)
Sauces with added meat or cheese	Sun-dried tomato pesto	
Sauces with added sugar or sucrose		

* Limit serving size (see page 25).

SNACKS

Bagels	Bananas	Almonds*
Candy	Dark chocolate * (70%	Applesauce
Cookies	cocoa)	(unsweetened)
Crackers	Ice cream (low-fat)	Canned peaches/pears in
Doughnuts	Most nuts*	juice or water
Flavoured gelatin (all	Popcorn (light,	Cottage cheese (1% or
varieties)	microwaveable)	fat-free)
French fries		Extra-low-fat cheese
Ice cream		(e.g., Laughing Cow
Melba toast		Light, Boursin Light)
Muffins (commercial)		Flavoured yogurt (non-
Popcorn (regular)		fat with sweetener)
Potato chips		Frozen yogurt (low-fat)
Pretzels		Hazelnuts*
Pudding		High-protein bars*
Raisins		Ice cream (1/2 cup, low-
Rice cakes/crackers		fat and no added
Sorbet		sugar)
Tortilla chips		Macadamia nuts*
Trail mix		Most fresh fruit
White bread		Most fresh/frozen
		vegetables
		Most seeds
		Pickles
		Soy nuts
		Sugar-free hard candies

SOUPS

All cream-based soups	Canned chicken noodle	Chunky bean and
Canned black bean	Canned lentil	vegetable soups (e.g.,
Canned green pea	Canned tomato	Campbell's Healthy
Canned puréed		Request, Healthy
vegetable		Choice)
Canned split pea		Homemade soups
		with green-light
		ingredients
		Miso soup

SPREADS & PRESERVES

All products that have		Fruit spreads (with fruit,
sugar as the first		not sugar, as the first
ingredient listed		ingredient)
		Marmite

*Limit serving size (see page 25).

SUGAR & SWEETENERS

Agave nectar	Fructose	Splenda
Corn syrup	Sugar alcohols	Stevia
Glucose		Sugar Twin
Honey		Sugar Twin Brown
Molasses		Sweet'N Low
Sugar (all types)		
Sugar Blend		
Splenda Brown		

VEGETABLES (FRESH/FROZEN)

Broad beans	Artichokes	Alfalfa sprouts
Coleslaw (commercial)	Beets	Asparagus
French fries	Corn	Beans (green/wax)
Hash browns	Pickles	Bell peppers
Parsnips	Potatoes (boiled)	Bok choy
Potatoes (instant)	Pumpkin	Broccoli
Potatoes (mashed or	Squash	Brussels sprouts
baked)	Sweet potatoes	Cabbage (all varieties)
Rutabaga	Yams	Carrots
Turnips		Cauliflower
		Celery
		Collard greens
		Cucumbers
		Eggplant
		Fennel
		Garlic
		Hearts of palm
		Kale
		Kohlrabi
		Leeks
		Lettuce
		Mushrooms
		Mustard greens
		Okra
		Olives*
		Onions
		Peas
		Peppers (hot)
		Potatoes (boiled, small, preferably new)
		Radicchio
		Radishes
		Rapini
		Salad greens (all varieties)
		Snow peas
		Spinach
		Swiss chard
		Tomatoes
		Zucchini

*Limit serving size (see page 25).

ACKNOWLEDGEMENTS

Sarah Brohman, who stepped in at the eleventh hour to edit my previous book, *The G.I. Diet Menopause Clinic*, to my great delight was available to edit this book. Again she was able to pull together a cohesive and compelling story out of the wealth of information provided by the diaries of the e-clinic members. I am most grateful.

Again, my thanks to Anne Collins, publisher of the Knopf Random Canada Publishing Group, who took a flyer on an unknown author eight years ago in publishing the original *G.I. Diet*, and for her encouragement over the subsequent eight titles in the series.

INDEX

sandwiches, 34–45
soups, 34

M

malignant melanoma, 135
malitol, 66
margarine, 14, 29, 31, 34, 37, 60–61
McDonald's, 109, 114, 150
meal plans
    plan A, 173–77
    plan B, 177–80
    plan C, 181–84
    plan D, 184–88
meal preparation, 65–67, 79
meat
    at breakfast, 28
    cooking methods, 38
    at dinner, 35
    G.I. Guide, 275
    at lunch, 32
    portion/serving size, 24, 73, 75
    at restaurants, 113
    soy alternative, *see* TVP
meat substitutes
    at dinner, 35
    at lunch, 32
medication, reducing, 4, 8, 19, 44, 86, 96, 122, 137
Mediterranean diet, 15, 80
men
    and andropause, 54, 102
    BMI, 23
    disease risk in, 101
    muscle mass, 143
    waist measurement, 45
    waist-to-hip ratio, 133
    weight gain in, 54, 55, 101, 102
    weight-waist measurement, 133
menopause, 5, 19, 54, 55, 102, 117, 133, 135
menstrual cycle, 19, 48, 117
Metformin, 90, 121, 122, 137
mesclun, 39
metabolism, 23, 55, 102, 120, 143, 126, 167
Mexican/Latin American restaurants, 112
microwave ovens, 67
mid-afternoon blues, 60, 88, *see also* , energy,
    flagging levels of
middle age, 3, 131, 132, 141–44, 151
milk, 31, 42

moderation, 42, 59, 69, 73, 75, 149, 167–68, 169
molasses, 66
monounsaturated fats, 14–15, 60
mood swings, 19
motivation, 4, 5, 6, 87–88, 122, 151, 158–59, 161
    tips, 86–88
mouth feel, 14, 97, 138
multiple myeloma, 135
muscle mass, 55, 143–44, 14\1

N

90 percent concept, 59, 115, 119, 121, 153, 169
Naturegg Break-Free, 32
Nestlé brand, 12
neurotransmitters, 15
non-Hodgkin lymphoma, 135
nuts, protein source, 16

O

oatmeal, 12, 30, 67, 68, *see also* steel-cut oatmeal
obesity
    and BMI, 21
    causes, ix, 11, 82
    health risks, 2–3, 54–55, 56–57, 103, 132, 133,
        134–35
    intl. comparisons, 72, 80
    statistics, 11
oils, *see also* specific oils
    at breakfast, 29
    at dinner, 37
    G.I. Guide, 273–74
    good/bad, 14–15
    at lunch, 34
olive oil, 14, 15, 65
Omega Pro, 32
omega-3 eggs, 68–69
omega-3 oils, 15, 38, 136
omelettes, 32
osteoarthritis, 145
overeating, 2–3, 59, 76, 78, 99
overweight, ix, 2–3, 11, 12, 21, 54–55, 133

P

packaged foods, 12
palm oil, 14
pancreas, 18
    cancer, 135
    cells, 2–3
pantry, 46, 149

RECIPE INDEX

Rick Gallop's bestselling *The G.I. Diet* was published in 2002 and quickly became the most successful Canadian diet book ever, with more than two million copies sold worldwide. It is currently available in twenty-three countries, in seventeen different languages. Gallop holds a Masters degree from Oxford University and was president and CEO of the Heart and Stroke Foundation of Ontario.